Contents

How To Use Springhouse Notes

Today, more than ever, nursing students face enormous time pressures. Nursing education has become more sophisticated, increasing the difficulties students have with studying efficiently and keeping pace.

The need for a comprehensive, well-designed series of study aids is great, which is why we've produced Springhouse Notes . . . to meet that need. Springhouse Notes provide essential course material in outline form, enabling the nursing student to study more effectively, improve understanding, achieve higher test scores, and get better grades.

Several key features appear throughout each book, making the information more accessible and easier to remember.
  • *Learning Objectives*. These objectives precede each section in the book to help the student evaluate knowledge before and after study.
  • *Key Points*. Highlighted in color throughout the book, these points provide a way to quickly review critical information. Key points may include:
  —a cardinal manifestation of a disorder
  —the most current or popular theory about a topic
  —a distinguishing characteristic of a disorder
  —the most important step of a process
  —a critical assessment component
  —a crucial nursing intervention
  —the most widely used or successful therapy or treatment
  • *Points to Remember*. This information, at the end of each section, summarizes the section in capsule form.
  • *Glossary*. Difficult, frequently used, or sometimes misunderstood terms are defined for the student at the end of each section.

Please note: Springhouse Notes are not intended for use as a primary information source. They should never substitute for class attendance, text-reading, or classroom note-taking.

The Fundamentals of Nursing Pharmacology

Learning Objectives

After studying this section, the reader should be able to:

● Explain how to use the nursing process when administering medications.

● Relate the contribution of federal drug legislation to the safety of medications in the United States.

● Identify the components of the pharmacokinetic phases of drug action.

● Discuss dosing schedules related to the pharmacokinetic actions of a drug.

● Define pharmacodynamics.

I. The Fundamentals of Nursing Pharmacology

A. The nursing process in medication administration

1. Assessment
   a. Ask the patient what prescription and nonprescription medications he is currently taking. How frequently does the patient take each medication? What is the purpose of each medication for this patient? What effects or side effects has the patient noticed from these medications?
   b. Find out if the patient has any food or drug allergies
   c. Take the patient's medical history
   d. Perform a physical examination, emphasizing the areas affected by the current medication before administering new medication
2. Nursing diagnosis
   a. Consists of a problem and its etiology
   b. Considers the patient's actual and potential problems
3. Planning
   a. Develop short-term and long-term goals from the nursing diagnosis, with input from the patient, if possible
   b. Use these goals as outcome criteria for evaluation
4. Implementation
   a. Administer medication according to the manufacturer's instructions
   b. Monitor the patient for therapeutic effects, where applicable, including serum drug levels and pertinent lab tests
   c. Assess the patient for side effects. Notify the physician and treat side effects as directed
   d. Consider patient teaching essential. Topics should include name of the drug, purpose, how and when to take the medication, methods of monitoring effectiveness (for example, monitoring blood pressure in patients on antihypertensives), other drugs that may interact with the prescribed medication, necessary dietary changes, side effects and what to do if they occur, signs and symptoms that should be brought to the physician's attention, and necessary follow-up procedures
   e. Include family members in patient teaching to encourage the patient and increase compliance
5. Evaluation
   a. Are the expected effects of the drug present? A physical examination and evaluation of lab test results may be necessary
   b. Is the patient experiencing side effects or interactions with other drugs or foods?
   c. Is the patient able to explain in his or her own words the information taught previously?
   d. Is the patient complying with the therapeutic regimen? If not, what are the reasons for noncompliance?
   e. Do you need to modify goals and interventions, based on your evaluation?

B. Drug legislation in the United States
1. Federal Food, Drug, and Cosmetic Act of 1906
   a. Empowered the federal government to enforce standards set by the United States Pharmacopeia (USP) and the National Formulary (NF)
   b. Required that drugs meet standards of strength and purity
   c. Required that the type and amount of narcotic be listed on the label of opiate mixtures
2. Sherley Amendment of 1912 prohibited use of fraudulent therapeutic claims
3. Food, Drug, and Cosmetic Act of 1938 stated that:
   a. Drugs and drug products must be tested for harmful effects
   b. Drug labels and literature must be complete and accurate, including dose, name and address of manufacturer, lists and amounts of ingredients that could be harmful, a warning if the drug might be habit-forming, directions for use, and contraindications
   c. Medical devices must be safe and effective
   d. Cosmetics must be safe
4. Durham-Humphrey Amendment of 1952
   a. Identified which drugs could be sold with or without a prescription
   b. Required that narcotics, hypnotics, habit-forming drugs, and potentially harmful drugs be refilled only with a new prescription and labeled as such
5. Kefauver-Harris or Drug Amendment of 1962
   a. Gave the Food and Drug Administration (FDA) more control over drug safety
   b. Allowed the FDA to evaluate the testing methods of drug manufacturers
   c. Required that drug manufacturers prove the effectiveness of a drug, not just the lack of toxicity
6. Controlled Substances Act or Comprehensive Drug Abuse Prevention Act of 1970
   a. Categorized controlled substances, such as narcotics, tranquilizers, barbiturates, and amphetamines, into five categories called schedules. These schedules are based on the drug's potential for abuse and on its medical effectiveness
   b. Limited how often a prescription for a controlled substance could be refilled

C. The five rights of medication administration
1. The right patient
2. The right medication
3. The right route
4. The right dose
5. The right time

D. Pharmacokinetics of drug action

1. Absorption: movement of a drug from its administration site across biological membranes into systemic circulation. The degree and rate of absorption depend on:
   a. The route
   b. The patient's age and disease state
   c. The drug's mechanism of absorption
   d. The potential interactions with other drugs or food
2. Distribution: movement of a drug from the systemic circulation into the tissue. Distribution may be affected by:
   a. The blood-brain barrier
   b. The rate of general circulation
   c. The blood supply of the target tissues
   d. The degree of vasoconstriction or vasodilation
   e. The degree of binding to plasma proteins: for example, albumin
3. Metabolism: alteration of the drug to a more active or less active form, usually in the liver. Metabolism may be affected by:
   a. Genetic factors
   b. Disease states
   c. Age
   d. The drug itself
4. Excretion: elimination of the drug from the circulation. Drugs may be excreted by:
   a. The kidney
   b. The liver
   c. The lungs
   d. Milk through breast-feeding
5. Dosing schedules: determined by the pharmacokinetics, including:
   a. Onset of action: the time when the drug's effects are first noticeable
   b. Peak concentration level: the time when the drug's actions are most potent
   c. Duration of action: the length of time the drug acts on the body
   d. Half-life: the point at which the drug's concentration in the plasma is decreased by one half

E. Pharmacodynamics involves the biochemical and physiologic effects of the drug. Pharmacodynamics includes:

1. Interaction with specific receptor sites
2. General interaction with cell metabolism
3. Alteration of the cellular environment

Points to Remember

The steps of the nursing process are assessment, diagnosis, planning, intervention, and evaluation. These steps should be used during the administration of all medications.

Federal drug legislation and regulations are designed to ensure the public's safety and to regulate the manufacture and sale of drugs.

The five rights of medication administration are the right patient, the right medication, the right route, the right dose, and the right time.

Pharmacokinetics of drug action include absorption, distribution, metabolism, and excretion (ADME).

Pharmacodynamics of drug action include interaction with specific receptor sites, general interaction with cell metabolism, and alteration of the cell's environment.

Glossary

Biological membrane—a layer of tissue separating one part from another; for example, skin, mucous membrane

Blood-brain barrier—a membrane between the circulating blood and the brain, preventing certain substances from reaching the brain or cerebrospinal fluid

Serum drug level—the amount of a drug present in the blood at a particular moment

United States Pharmacopeia—compendium of drugs and their preparation issued every year by a national committee of experts; adopted as U.S. standard in 1906

The Patient Requiring an Autonomic Nervous System Drug

Learning Objectives

After studying this section, the reader should be able to:

- Describe the relationship between the physiologic responses of the autonomic nervous system and the drugs that affect it.

- Explain the general principles of action of parasympathetic nervous system agents, neuromuscular blocking agents, and sympathetic nervous system agents.

- List the indications for the various types of parasympathetic and sympathetic nervous system agents.

- Identify the nursing implications during assessment, implementation, and evaluation of the patient receiving each class of drugs affecting the autonomic nervous system.

- Discuss appropriate patient teaching for the patient receiving each class of drugs affecting the autonomic nervous system.

II. The Patient Requiring an Autonomic Nervous System Drug

A. Parasympathetic nervous system agents: general information

1. Mechanism of action: mimic or inhibit parasympathetic activity by activating or inhibiting receptors normally activated by acetylcholine
2. Indications
   a. Parasympathomimetic and cholinergic agents: to treat glaucoma and to stimulate bladder and intestinal function
   b. Acetylcholinesterase inhibitors: to treat myasthenia gravis and glaucoma, and to prevent or treat postoperative paralytic ileus
   c. Parasympatholytic and anticholinergic agents: as preoperative medication; to treat Parkinson's disease, GI spasms, motion sickness, and enuresis; to reverse heart block; as mydriatic agents
   d. Neuromuscular-blocking agents: to induce skeletal muscle relaxation in order to facilitate general anesthesia
3. Contraindications: see specific information
4. Side effects: see specific information
5. Interactions
   a. Parasympathomimetic, cholinergic agents and acetylcholinesterase inhibitors potentiate each other
   b. Parasympatholytic and anticholinergic agents have additive effects with other anticholinergic agents
6. Nursing implications: see specific information
7. Patient teaching: see specific information

B. Parasympathomimetic and cholinergic agents: specific information

1. Indications
   a. Nonobstructive urinary retention, neurogenic bladder, and adynamic ileus (bethanechol)
   b. Glaucoma (pilocarpine)
2. Contraindications: avoid use in patients with possible urinary or GI obstruction or an enlarged prostate
3. Side effects
   a. Flushing, sweating, increased salivation, abdominal cramps, nausea, vomiting, diarrhea
   b. Headache, hypotension
4. Interactions: atropine-like drugs inhibit the action of these drugs
5. Nursing implications
   a. Assessment: assess patient's GI or urinary status; monitor for drug toxicity
   b. Implementation: administer atropine as the antidote for toxicity
   c. Evaluation: base on increased bladder or intestinal tone and function, or decreased intraocular pressure
6. Patient teaching: include instruction on the proper administration of eye drops, as needed

7. Drug examples
   a. Bethanechol (Urecholine)
   b. Pilocarpine (Isopto Carpine, Mi-pilo, Pilocar)

C. Acetylcholinesterase inhibitors: specific information

1. Indications
   a. To diagnose myasthenia gravis (edrophonium)
   b. To treat myasthenia gravis (neostigmine, pyridostigmine)
   c. To prevent or treat postoperative ileus (neostigmine)
   d. To manage cholinergic excess, including treatment of overdose of tricyclic antidepressants, and glaucoma (physostigmine)
2. Contraindications: avoid use in patients with possible urinary or GI obstructions
3. Side effects
   a. Muscarinic: nausea, vomiting, diarrhea, increased salivation, dyspnea, diaphoresis, miosis, bradycardia, hypotension
   b. Nicotinic: muscle cramps, hypertension, fatigue, weakness, respiratory depression, paralysis
4. Interactions: parenteral neostigmine antagonizes nondepolarizing neuromuscular blocking agents (for example, tubocurarine) and prolongs actions of depolarizing muscle relaxants (for example, succinylcholine)
5. Nursing implications
   a. Assessment: assess neuromuscular status
   b. Implementation: administer atropine as the antidote for toxicity
   c. Evaluation: base on improvement of neuromuscular symptoms and strength without cholinergic symptoms
6. Patient teaching: see Section VIII
7. Drug examples
   a. Edrophonium (Tensilon)
   b. Neostigmine (Prostigmin)
   c. Pyridostigmine (Mestinon)
   d. Physostigmine (Antilirium, Eserine)

D. Parasympatholytic and anticholinergic agents: specific information

1. Indications
   a. To treat bradyarrhythmias: atropine
   b. To prevent nausea and vomiting from motion sickness: scopolamine
   c. To treat peptic ulcer and bowel spasms: propantheline and glycopyrrolate
   d. To manage dyskinesias (parkinsonism): benztropine and trihexylphenidyl
   e. To produce mydriasis: atropine
   f. To produce a preoperative decrease in saliva and bronchial secretions: atropine, scopolamine, glycopyrrolate

2. Contraindications: narrow-angle glaucoma and severe hemorrhage, uncontrolled tachycardia, urinary or GI tract obstructions
3. Side effects
   a. Ophthalmic: photophobia, blurred vision, conjunctivitis
   b. Systemic: tachycardia, dry mouth, urinary hesitancy, constipation
4. Interactions
   a. Additive anticholinergic effects occur with similar-acting drugs
   b. Antacids may decrease absorption of anticholinergics
5. Nursing implications
   a. Assessment: assess patient for relief of symptoms and potential side effects
   b. Implementation: place transdermal scopolamine system behind the ear at least 4 hours before travel
   c. Evaluation: base on resolution of symptoms without severe side effects
6. Patient teaching
   a. Teach patient to administer eye drops
   b. Discuss methods to minimize dry mouth and constipation
   c. Instruct patient not to take over-the-counter drugs without consulting physician or pharmacist
7. Drug examples
   a. Atropine
   b. Scopolamine (Transderm Scop)
   c. Propantheline (Pro-Banthine)
   d. Glycopyrrolate (Robinul)

E. Neuromuscular blocking agents: specific information
  1. Mechanism of action
     a. Prevent activation and depolarization of muscle fiber by acetylcholine (tubocurarine)
     b. Mimic acetylcholine, depolarize the neuromuscular junction and block further depolarization (succinylcholine)
  2. Drug examples
     a. Tubocurarine (Tubadil, Tubarine)
     b. Succinylcholine (Anectine)

F. Sympathetic nervous system agents: general information
  1. Mechanism of action: mimic or inhibit sympathetic activity by activating or inhibiting receptors normally activated by norepinephrine
  2. Indications
     a. Sympathomimetics or adrenergic agents: allergic reactions, asthma, hypotension, cardiac arrest, nasal decongestion, bronchodilation
     b. Alpha-adrenergic blocking agents: peripheral vascular disorders, Raynaud's disease, vascular headaches, adrenergic excess (for example, pheochromocytoma)

      c. Beta-adrenergic blocking agents: hypertension, angina, tachyarrhythmias; migraine headache prophylaxis; prevention of myocardial infarction, glaucoma, acute anxiety reaction

  3. Contraindications: see specific information

  4. Side effects: see specific information

  5. Interactions

      a. Sympathomimetic and adrenergic agents have additive effects with other adrenergic drugs

      b. Adrenergic blocking agents have additive effects with other antiadrenergic agents

  6. Nursing implications: see specific information

  7. Patient teaching: see specific information

G. Sympathomimetic and adrenergic agents: specific information

  1. Indications

      a. Epinephrine: bronchodilation in asthma or allergic reactions; cardiac stimulation in cardiac arrest; mydriasis; combined with local anesthetics for longer duration

      b. Isoproterenol: cardiac stimulation and bronchodilation

      c. Norepinephrine: cardiac stimulation and increase in blood pressure through vasoconstriction

      d. Dopamine: increased blood pressure and cardiac output via positive inotropic action, increased renal and mesenteric blood flow

      e. Dobutamine: increase in myocardial force and cardiac output

  2. Contraindications and precautions

      a. Narrow-angle glaucoma (epinephrine)

      b. Tachyarrhythmias (dopamine, isoproterenol)

  3. Side effects: dysrhythmias, tachycardia, angina, restlessness

  4. Interactions: epinephrine, norepinephrine, and isoproterenol antagonize the effects of beta-blocking agents

  5. Nursing implications

      a. Assessment: assess vital signs, EKG, hemodynamic parameters, lung sounds, and urine output

      b. Implementation: correct hypovolemia before infusing dopamine or norepinephrine. If either of these infusions extravasate, infiltrate skin with phentolamine and normal saline solution

      c. Evaluation: base on improved vital signs, hemodynamic parameters, and urine output, and a decrease in bronchospasm

  6. Patient teaching

      a. Explain the drugs' purposes when used in a hospital setting

      b. Instruct patient on correct administration of inhalation agents

  7. Drug examples

      a. Epinephrine (Adrenalin, Primatene, Sus-Phrine)

      b. Isoproterenol (Isuprel)

    c. Norepinephrine (Levophed)
    d. Dopamine (Intropin)
    e. Dobutamine (Dobutrex)

H. Alpha-adrenergic blocking agents: specific information
  1. Indications
    a. To control Raynaud's disease: phenoxybenzamine
    b. To diagnose and treat hypertension from pheochromocytoma and to treat extravasation of vasopressors: phentolamine
    c. To treat vascular headaches: ergotamine
  2. Contraindications: myocardial infarction, pregnancy
  3. Side effects
    a. Nasal congestion, tachycardia, dizziness, GI irritation, hypotension, miosis: phenoxybenzamine, phentolamine
    b. Ergotism, which includes numbness, tingling of digits, weakness, blindness: ergotamine
  4. Interactions: phenoxybenzamine potentiates hypotensive effects of antihypertensives
  5. Nursing implications
    a. Assessment: monitor blood pressure with phenoxybenzamine and phentolamine
    b. Implementation: withhold all antihypertensive agents during phentolamine test
    c. Evaluation: base on improved peripheral circulation in Raynaud's disease; decreased blood pressure in pheochromocytoma; relief of vascular headache
  6. Patient teaching
    a. Tell patient to change positions slowly to minimize orthostatic hypotension
    b. Inform patient that phenoxybenzamine may require 1 week of therapy before results are evident
    c. Explain procedure for phentolamine test
    d. Instruct patient with vascular headaches to take drug at onset of pain and lie down in a dark, quiet room
  7. Drug examples
    a. Phenoxybenzamine (Dibenzyline)
    b. Phentolamine (Regitine)
    c. Ergotamine tartate (Gynergen), with caffeine (Cafergot)

I. Beta-adrenergic blocking agents: specific information
  1. Indications
    a. Hypertension: atenolol, labetalol, metoprolol, nadolol, propranolol, timolol
    b. Angina: atenolol, metoprolol, nadolol, propranolol
    c. Type III dysrhythmias: propranolol
    d. Myocardial infarction prophylaxis: metoprolol, propranolol, timolol

     e. Vascular headache prophylaxis: propranolol

     f. Glaucoma: (locally applied) timolol

2. Contraindications: congestive heart failure, bronchospasm, bradyarrhythmias, heart block

3. Side effects

     a. Bradycardia, bronchospasm, dysrhythmias

     b. Nausea, vomiting, diarrhea

     c. Increased sensitivity to cold

4. Interactions

     a. Additive myocardial depression and bradycardia with agents that have similar effects (digitalis glycosides, antiarrhythmics, calcium channel blockers)

     b. Increased potential for hypoglycemia; may alter insulin needs

5. Nursing implications

     a. Assessment: assess heart rate; hold drug and notify physician if less than 50 beats/minute, or according to hospital policy

     b. Evaluation: base on a decrease in blood pressure and angina; resolution of dysrhythmias; prevention of myocardial infarction and vascular headaches

6. Patient teaching

     a. Teach patient to monitor pulse and blood pressure

     b. Encourage patient to comply with other therapy for hypertension (weight reduction, smoking cessation, low-sodium diet, regular exercise, stress management)

     c. Patient should carry identification describing disease and drug regimen

7. Drug examples

     a. Atenolol (Tenormin)

     b. Labetalol (Normodyne, Trandate)

     c. Metoprolol (Lopressor)

     d. Nadolol (Corgard)

     e. Propranolol (Inderal)

     f. Timolol (Blocadren)

Points to Remember

Drugs acting on the autonomic nervous system either stimulate or inhibit the neurotransmitters, norepinephrine and acetylcholine, or their receptor sites. Stimulation of norepinephrine results in a response similar to the sympathetic nervous system. Stimulation of acetylcholine mimics a parasympathetic response.

Drugs that affect the sympathetic nervous system activate or suppress alpha-, beta$_1$-, and/or beta$_2$-receptor sites.

Alpha adrenergic stimulation causes vasoconstriction, resulting in hypertension. Drugs that inhibit alpha-adrenergic receptors cause vasodilation and can be used to treat hypertensive crisis.

Drugs that stimulate beta$_1$ receptors increase cardiac contractility and heart rate and accelerate atrioventricular conduction in the heart. Inhibition of the beta$_1$ receptors causes slowing of the heart rate and decreased force of cardiac contraction and can be used to treat angina or hypertension.

Stimulation of the beta$_2$ receptors causes bronchodilation and peripheral vasodilation. Drugs that inhibit the beta$_2$ receptors may cause bronchoconstriction and peripheral vasoconstriction.

Glossary

Acetylcholinesterase inhibitor—a drug that blocks the action of acetylcholinesterase, an enzyme that terminates the effects of acetylcholine. These drugs increase parasympathetic activity

Adrenergic blocking agent—a drug that interferes with the transmission of nerve impulses to adrenergic receptors, allowing for a parasympathetic response

Parasympatholytic—a drug that blocks the effects of the parasympathetic nervous system, allowing for a sympathetic response

Parasympathomimetic (cholinergic)—a drug that mimics the effects of the parasympathetic nervous system

Sympathomimetic (adrenergic)—a drug that mimics the effects of the sympathetic nervous system

The Patient Requiring Pain Medication

Learning Objectives

After studying this section, the reader should be able to:

● Describe the mechanism of action of narcotic analgesics, non-narcotic analgesics and narcotic antagonists.

● List the nursing responsibilities for pain management with analgesic drugs.

● Discuss nursing measures that may be used to enhance the therapeutic response to analgesics.

● Discuss appropriate patient teaching for patients receiving narcotic and non-narcotic analgesics.

III. The Patient Requiring Pain Medication

A. Pain medication: general information

1. Mechanism of action
   a. Narcotic analgesics: bind to opiate receptors in the central nervous system (CNS), altering the perception of and emotional response to pain. Controlled substances
   b. Narcotic agonists/antagonists: compete for opiate receptors in the brain, altering the perception of and response to pain, and prevent the binding of narcotic analgesics to these sites. Most are controlled substances
   c. Narcotic antagonists: competitively block the effects of narcotics, without producing analgesic effects
   d. Non-narcotic analgesics: act peripherally to prevent the formation of prostaglandins in inflamed tissue, inhibiting the stimulation of pain receptors. Also, inhibit prostaglandin synthesis in the CNS and stimulate peripheral vasodilation to cause antipyresis
2. Indications: pain (except for narcotic antagonists). The level of pain and response to previous treatments determine the type of analgesic needed
3. Contraindications: see specific information
4. Side effects: nausea and vomiting (except for naloxone and acetaminophen)
5. Interactions: see specific information
6. Nursing implications
   a. Assessment: assess level of pain before administration and at the medication's peak concentration level
   b. Implementation: use alternate methods of pain management to enhance the effects of the medication; for example, positioning, relaxation, imaging, distraction, massage
   c. Evaluation: base on decrease in or relief of pain without serious side effects
7. Patient teaching
   a. Explain the purpose of the medication; this can enhance the analgesic effect
   b. Instruct patient how and when the medication should be taken for maximum effectiveness. Explain procedure for medications to be given as needed

B. Narcotic analgesics and narcotic agonists/antagonists: specific information

1. Indications
   a. Pain unresponsive to non-narcotic analgesics
   b. Adjunct to anesthesia (meperidine, morphine, butorphanol, nalbuphine, pentazocine)
   c. Cough (codeine, hydromorphone)
   d. Acute pulmonary edema (morphine)

2. Contraindications and precautions
   a. Caution should be used in head injury, hepatic or renal disease, or CNS depression
   b. Elderly or debilitated patients may require decreased dosages
   c. Use of narcotic agonists/antagonists in patients physically dependent on narcotics may cause withdrawal symptoms
3. Side effects
   a. Respiratory depression, orthostatic hypotension
   b. Sedation, dizziness, lightheadedness, dysphoria
   c. Constipation
   d. Tolerance, physical and psychological dependence
4. Interactions
   a. Additive CNS depression occurs with alcohol, antihistamines, and sedative/hypnotics
   b. Narcotic agonists/antagonists may cause withdrawal symptoms in patients physically dependent on narcotic analgesics
   c. Concurrent administration with non-narcotic analgesics may enhance pain relief because they act at different sites
5. Nursing implications
   a. Assessment: assess blood pressure, pulse and respiratory status before and periodically after administration
   b. Implementation: administer before pain is severe for better analgesic effect. Regular administration may be more effective than doses as needed. Prolonged use may lead to dependence and tolerance, but this should not prevent patient from receiving adequate analgesia. Patients receiving narcotics for medical reasons rarely develop psychological dependence. They may require progressively higher doses to relieve pain with long-term therapy. Drugs should be discontinued gradually after long-term use to prevent withdrawal symptoms. Naloxone is the antidote
6. Patient teaching
   a. Tell patient to take oral doses with food to minimize GI irritation
   b. Instruct patient to change position slowly to minimize orthostatic hypotension
   c. Warn patient to avoid activities requiring alertness until effects of drug are known
   d. Discuss ways to minimize dry mouth and constipation
7. Drug examples
   a. Morphine sulfate (MS)
   b. Hyrdomorphone (Dilaudid)
   c. Meperidine (Demerol)
   d. Codeine
   e. Oxycodone (Percodan, Percocet, Tylox)
   f. Propoxyphene (Darvon, Darvocet)
   g. Buprenorphine (Buprenex)

    h. Butorphanol (Stadol)
    i.   Nalbuphine (Nubain)
    j.   Pentazocine (Talwin, Talwin NX)

C. Narcotic antagonists: specific information
  1. Indications: used to reverse CNS and respiratory depression in narcotic overdosage
  2. Contraindications and precautions: use with caution in narcotic-dependent patients; may cause severe withdrawal symptoms
  3. Side effects: hypotension, hypertension, dysrhythmias
  4. Interactions: reverse effects of narcotics
  5. Nursing implications
    a. Assessment: assess respiratory status, blood pressure, pulse, and level of consciousness until narcotic wears off. Repeat doses may be necessary if effect of narcotic outlasts the effect of the narcotic antagonist
    b. Implementation: remember that narcotic antagonists reverse analgesia along with respiratory depression. Titrate dose accordingly and monitor pain level
    c. Evaluation: base on improved respiratory status and alertness without significant pain. Lack of marked improvement indicates that symptoms are caused by CNS depressants other than narcotics, or by a disease process
  6. Drug example: naloxone (Narcan)

D. Non-narcotic analgesics: specific information
  1. Indications
    a. Mild to moderate pain: acetaminophen, aspirin, diflunisal, ibuprofen, naproxen
    b. Fever: acetaminophen, aspirin, ibuprofen
    c. Inflammation: aspirin, naproxen
    d. Arthritis: aspirin, diflunisal, ibuprofen, naproxen, piroxicam, sulindac
    e. Dysmenorrhea: ibuprofen, naproxen
    f. Prevention of transient ischemic attacks and myocardial infarction: aspirin
  2. Contraindications and precautions
    a. All, except acetaminophen, are contraindicated in pregnancy
    b. Aspirin is contraindicated in bleeding disorders or GI ulcers
    c. Hypersensitivity to aspirin is a contraindication to the entire class, except acetaminophen
    d. Caution should be used in patients with asthma or nasal polyps
  3. Side effects
    a. GI pain and upset, nausea, vomiting, diarrhea, heartburn
    b. Dizziness, headache, tinnitus

    c. Acetaminophen: hypersensitivity (laryngeal edema, skin rash, fever, angioneurotic edema, mucosal lesions)

4. Interactions
    a. Nonsteroidal anti-inflammatory agents may prolong bleeding time and increase the effects of oral anticoagulants
    b. Use of aspirin with other nonsteroidal anti-inflammatory agents may increase GI effects and decrease effectiveness
    c. Chronic use of acetaminophen with nonsteroidal anti-inflammatory agents may increase the chance of renal side effects
    d. Concurrent administration with narcotic analgesics may enhance pain relief
    e. Use of nonsteroidal anti-inflammatory agents with alcohol may increase GI side effects

5. Nursing implications: administer before meals for more rapid effect or with meals to minimize GI irritation

6. Patient teaching
    a. Instruct patient to inform physician or dentist of medication regimen before treatment or surgery
    b. Advise patient that the Centers for Disease Control warns against giving aspirin to children or adolescents with influenza, varicella (chicken pox), or viral illness because of a possible association with Reye's syndrome

7. Drug examples
    a. Acetaminophen (Tylenol, Datril, Tempra)
    b. Aspirin (ASA, acetylsalicylic acid)
    c. Diflunisal (Dolobid)
    d. Ibuprofen (Motrin, Nuprin, Advil, Haltran, Medipren, Trendar, Rufen)
    e. Naproxen (Naprosyn); naproxen sodium (Anaprox)
    f. Piroxicam (Feldene)
    g. Sulindac (Clinoril)

Points to Remember

Narcotic analgesics and narcotic agonists/antagonists act on the central nervous system to alter the perception of and the emotional response to pain. Non-narcotic analgesics act on the peripheral nervous system to prevent the formation of prostaglandins, which stimulate pain receptors. Combining adequate amounts of these two types of analgesics may provide more effective pain relief than either one alone.

Assessment of the patient's level of pain before administration of an analgesic and again at the peak of its effect is necessary for effective pain management.

Analgesics are more effective if they are given regularly, before pain becomes severe.

The possibility of physical or psychological dependence should not prevent the patient from receiving adequate pain medication. Patients receiving narcotics for acute pain rarely develop psychological dependence. Progressively higher doses may be required to provide pain relief during long-term therapy.

Glossary

Antipyresis—reduction of fever

Controlled substances—depressant or stimulant drugs and drugs of abuse or potential abuse whose distribution and use are controlled under the Comprehensive Drug Abuse Prevention Act of 1970

Dysphoria—feelings of unrest, restlessness, and anxiety

Narcotic agonists/antagonists—drugs that provide pain relief by competing with opiate receptors in the brain. These drugs also prevent the binding of narcotic analgesics to opiate receptors and cause withdrawal symptoms in patients physically dependent on narcotics

The Patient Requiring an Anesthetic

Learning Objectives

After studying this section, the reader should be able to:

- Describe the mechanism of action of general and local anesthetics.

- Compare the effects of general and local anesthesia on the patient undergoing surgery.

- List nursing responsibilities for patients receiving general and local anesthesia.

- Discuss appropriate patient teaching for patients receiving general and local anesthesia.

IV. The Patient Requiring an Anesthetic

A. General anesthesia: general information
  1. Mechanism of action: causes progressive, reversible central nervous system (CNS) depression
  2. Indications: to prevent pain during surgery
  3. Contraindications and precautions: use with caution in patients with unstable cardiovascular or respiratory systems
  4. Side effects: see specific information
  5. Interactions: additive CNS depression with similar-acting drugs
  6. Nursing implications
      a. Assessment: assess patient's cardiovascular, respiratory, and renal status, and level of consciousness before and after surgery. Determine any allergies the patient may have
      b. Evaluation: base on pain and major side effects throughout surgery
  7. Patient teaching
      a. Discuss with the patient what to expect during the surgical experience
      b. Explain that no food and fluids will be allowed for at least 8 hours before surgery

B. Rapid-acting barbiturates: specific information
  1. Indications: induction and maintenance of anesthesia
  2. Drug examples
      a. Thiopental sodium (Pentothal)
      b. Methohexital sodium (Brevital)

C. Inhalation anesthetics: specific information
  1. Indications: maintenance of anesthesia
  2. Side effects: postanesthesia nausea and vomiting
  3. Drug examples
      a. Nitrous oxide
      b. Halothane (Fluothane)
      c. Methoxyflurane (Penthrane)
      d. Enflurane (Ethrane)
      e. Isoflurane (Forane)

D. Neuromuscular blocking agents (see Section II): specific information
  1. Mechanism of action
      a. Prevent activation and depolarization of muscle fiber by acetylcholine (tubocurarine, pancuronium bromide, atracurium)
      b. Mimic acetylcholine, depolarize the neuromuscular junction, and block further depolarization (succinylcholine)
  2. Indications: deep muscle relaxation and paralysis during surgery
  3. Drug examples
      a. Tubocurarine (Tubadil, Tubarine)
      b. Pancuronium bromide (Pavulon)

    c. Atracurium (Tracrium)
    d. Succinylcholine (Anectine)

E. Analgesics: specific information
1. Indications: induction of anesthesia and pain relief
2. Drug example: fentanyl (Sublimaze)

F. Neuroleptanesthesia: specific information
1. Mechanism of action: produces dissociation from the environment during induction (ketamine, droperidol) and produces pain relief and sedation (fentanyl)
2. Indications: short surgical procedures
3. Side effects: disturbing dreams or hallucinations during emergence from anesthesia (ketamine)
4. Nursing implications: patients receiving droperidol/fentanyl (Innovar) during surgery must have all doses of analgesics and other CNS depressants reduced by one third to one half for 8 hours following anesthesia
5. Drug examples
    a. Ketamine (Ketalar)
    b. Droperidol (Inapsine)
    c. Droperidol/fentanyl (Innovar)

G. Local anesthesia: general information
1. Mechanism of action: stabilizes the nerve cell membranes to sodium and potassium exchange, blocking the conduction of impulses in nerve fibers
2. Indications: surgery without CNS depression
3. Contraindications and precautions: elderly or debilitated patients are at a greater risk for developing toxicity
4. Side effects: toxicity, dysrhythmias, bradycardia, hypotension
5. Interactions: epinephrine may be combined with local anesthetics to slow drug absorption and prolong anesthetic effect
6. Nursing implications: assess patient's movement and sensation following surgery. Onset affects ability to sense cold, warmth, pain, touch, and then affects motor function. Sensation returns in reverse order
7. Patient teaching: prepare patient for lack of sensation after surgery
8. Drug examples
    a. Lidocaine hydrochloride (Xylocaine)
    b. Bupivacaine hydrochloride (Marcaine)
    c. Tetracaine hydrochloride (Pontocaine)

Points to Remember

Anesthetics should be used with caution in the patient with an unstable cardiovascular or respiratory system.

Neuroleptanesthesia is for short surgical procedures.

The patient receiving droperidol/fentanyl (Innovar) during surgery must have all doses of analgesics and other CNS depressants reduced by one third to one half for 8 hours following anesthesia.

Local anesthetics stabilize the nerve cell membranes to sodium and potassium exchange, thus blocking the conduction of impulses in nerve fibers.

Glossary

Acetylcholine—neurotransmitter at the neuromuscular junction

Depolarization—neutralization of electrical polarity of cell membrane

Epinephrine—hormone secreted by the adrenal gland; powerful stimulator of the sympathetic nervous system; called adrenaline by British

Hypotension—blood pressure below normal

The Patient Requiring a Central Nervous System Stimulant

Learning Objectives

After studying this section, the reader should be able to:

- Describe the mechanism of action of central nervous system stimulants.

- Name common side effects of central nervous system stimulants.

- List nursing responsibilities for the patient receiving central nervous system stimulants.

- Discuss appropriate patient teaching for the patient receiving central nervous system stimulants.

V. The Patient Requiring a Central Nervous System Stimulant

A. Central nervous system (CNS) stimulants: general information

1. Mechanism of action: increase levels of neurotransmitters in the CNS, causing CNS and respiratory stimulation, dilated pupils, increased motor activity and mental alertness, brighter spirits, and a diminished sense of fatigue
2. Indications
   a. Narcolepsy
   b. Adjunctive treatment to manage attention deficit disorder
   c. Former use as adjunctive treatment to manage exogenous obesity
   d. Respiratory stimulation after anesthesia (doxapram)
3. Contraindications and precautions
   a. Contraindicated in glaucoma and severe cardiovascular disease
   b. Avoid use during pregnancy or lactation, or in patients with psychotic personalities
4. Side effects
   a. Acute (toxicity): restlessness, tremor, irritability, insomnia, hypotension, dysrhythmias, angina, cardiovascular collapse
   b. Chronic: marked weight loss, fatigue, irritability, depression
5. Interactions
   a. Additive sympathomimetic effects occur with similar drugs
   b. Changes in urinary pH may alter effectiveness
6. Nursing implications
   a. Assessment: assess patient's behavior and monitor growth in children on long-term therapy. Assess respiratory status and arterial blood gas measurements in patients receiving doxapram
   b. Implementation: remember that most CNS stimulants are controlled substances; amphetamines may cause dependence and abuse
   c. Evaluation: base on increased activity and alertness, diminished fatigue, and brighter spirits in patients with narcolepsy. In children with hyperkinetic syndrome, a calming effect with decreased hyperactivity and prolonged attention span may be seen in 3 to 4 weeks. Check for improved respiratory status and arterial blood gas measurements in patients receiving doxapram
7. Patient teaching
   a. Instruct the patient to take the last dose before 6 p.m. to prevent insomnia
   b. Warn the patient to avoid beverages containing caffeine while taking this drug

B. Central nervous system stimulants: specific information
  1. Indications
     a. Narcolepsy (methylphenidate, amphetamines, pemoline)
     b. Attention deficit disorders (methylphenidate, pemoline, amphetamines)
     c. Former use as adjunctive treatment of exogenous obesity (amphetamines)
  2. Drug examples
     a. Methylphenidate (Ritalin)
     b. Pemoline (Cylert)
     c. Amphetamine (Biphetamine); dextroamphetamine (Dexedrine)
     d. Doxapram (Dopram)

Points to Remember

Children on long-term CNS stimulant therapy should have their growth monitored regularly.

Most CNS stimulants are controlled substances.

Amphetamines may cause dependence and abuse.

CNS stimulants may have a calming effect on children with hyperkinetic syndrome in 3 to 4 weeks.

CNS stimulants should be administered before 6 p.m. to prevent insomnia.

Glossary

Arterial blood gas measurements—the amount of oxygen and carbon dioxide in arterial blood

Attention deficit disorder—syndrome that may include decreased attention span; increased impulsivity and emotional lability; impairment in such areas as perception, language, memory, and motor skills; and, usually, hyperactivity

Hyperkinetic—hyperactive

Narcolepsy—a chronic ailment consisting of recurrent attacks of drowsiness and sleep. The patient is unable to control the spells but is easily awakened

The Patient with a Convulsive Disorder

Learning Objectives

After studying this section, the reader should be able to:

- Explain the general mechanism of action of the anticonvulsant drugs.

- Identify the nursing implications during assessment, implementation, and evaluation of the patient receiving anticonvulsant therapy.

- Discuss appropriate patient teaching for the patient receiving anticonvulsant therapy.

- List the most common side effects of the various anticonvulsant drugs.

VI. The Patient with a Convulsive Disorder

A. Anticonvulsants: general information

1. Mechanism of action: depress abnormal neuronal discharges and prevent the spread of seizure activity
2. Indications: control of seizures (for example, from epilepsy)
3. Contraindications and precautions
   a. Watch for hypersensitivity
   b. Use cautiously during pregnancy
4. Side effects: drowsiness
5. Interactions
   a. Anticonvulsants potentiate central nervous system (CNS) depressants and alcohol
   b. Tricyclic antidepressants and phenothiazines lower the seizure threshold and decrease effectiveness of anticonvulsants
6. Nursing implications
   a. Assessment: assess location, duration, and characteristics of seizure activity
   b. Implementation: do not give orally with milk or antacids; this will impair absorption. May give with food to decrease GI irritation. Implement seizure precautions
   c. Evaluation: base on cessation of seizure activity without side effects
7. Patient teaching
   a. Instruct patient not to discontinue medication without consulting physician, as this may cause seizures
   b. Warn patient not to drink alcohol with this medication
   c. Urge patient to use caution when driving or during activities requiring alertness until effects of drug are known
   d. Tell patient to carry identification describing disease and drug regimen

B. Hydantoins: specific information

1. Indications
   a. Tonic-clonic (grand mal) seizures
   b. Complex partial seizures
   c. Dysrhythmias (phenytoin)
2. Side effects
   a. Gingival hyperplasia
   b. Toxicity: therapeutic blood levels should be monitored. Signs and symptoms of toxicity include diplopia, nystagmus, ataxia, and drowsiness
3. Interactions: phenytoin may alter the effect of oral anticoagulants
4. Nursing implications
   a. Assessment: monitor patient for signs of toxicity
   b. Implementation: dilute phenytoin (Dilantin) in normal saline solution when administering it intravenously; dextrose solutions will cause a precipitate. Administer phenytoin slowly

5. Patient teaching
   a. Emphasize the importance of good oral hygiene and regular dental examinations to prevent gingival hyperplasia
   b. Tell patient to consult physician or pharmacist before changing drug brands because brands may have different effects
6. Drug example: phenytoin (Dilantin)

C. Barbiturates: specific information
1. Indications
   a. Tonic-clonic (grand mal) seizures
   b. Partial seizures
   c. Insomnia
   d. Adjunct to anesthesia
2. Side effects: dizziness
3. Interactions: primidone decreases phenytoin level
4. Drug examples
   a. Phenobarbital (Luminal)
   b. Primidone (Mysoline)

D. Benzodiazepines: specific information
1. Indications
   a. Absence seizures (clonazepam)
   b. Status epilepticus (diazepam)
   c. Anxiety (diazepam)
   d. Skeletal muscle spasms (diazepam)
2. Adverse reactions and side effects
   a. Ataxia
   b. Respiratory and cardiovascular depression (diazepam I.V.)
3. Drug examples
   a. Clonazepam (Klonopin)
   b. Diazepam (Valium)

E. Succinimides: specific information
1. Indications: absence seizures
2. Side effects: anorexia, nausea, vomiting
3. Drug example: ethosuximide (Zarontin)

F. Miscellaneous anticonvulsants: specific information
1. Indications
   a. Carbamazepine: tonic-clonic seizures, simple and complex partial seizures, trigeminal neuralgia
   b. Valproic acid: absence seizures
2. Drug examples
   a. Carbamazepine (Tegretol)
   b. Valproic acid (Depakene)

Points to Remember

Anticonvulsants are used to treat various types of epileptic seizures.

The most common side effect of anticonvulsants is drowsiness.

Nursing assessment includes noting the location, duration, and characteristics of seizure activity.

Nursing implementation includes using seizure precautions.

Patients should be taught the importance of compliance with this medication regimen because sudden cessation may lead to status epilepticus.

Glossary

Ataxia—incoordination of voluntary muscle action, particularly in activities such as walking or reaching for objects

Epilepsy—a disorder characterized by convulsive seizures or disturbances of consciousness, or both, from electrical activity disturbance in the brain

Gingival hyperplasia—an overgrowth of gum tissue

Nystagmus—constant, involuntary movement of the eyes

Status epilepticus—a rapid succession of seizures without intervals of consciousness. This constitutes a medical emergency

The Patient with Parkinson's Disease

Learning Objectives

After studying this section, the reader should be able to:

- Explain the pathophysiology of Parkinson's disease and how it relates to the drugs used to treat it.

- Develop a plan to assess the patient with Parkinson's disease for the effectiveness of the medication regimen.

- List common side effects of medications for Parkinson's disease.

- Discuss appropriate patient teaching for the patient receiving medication for Parkinson's disease.

VII. The Patient with Parkinson's Disease

A. Antiparkinsonian agents: general information

1. Mechanism of action: restore the natural balance of the neurotransmitters acetylcholine and dopamine in the central nervous system (CNS). The deficiency of dopamine causes excessive cholinergic activity
2. Indications: used to treat Parkinson's disease
3. Contraindications: do not use anticholinergics with patients who have narrow-angle glaucoma
4. Adverse reactions and side effects: see specific information
5. Interactions: see specific information
6. Nursing implications
   a. Assessment: assess patient for symptoms of parkinsonism (rigidity, tremors, akinesia)
   b. Implementation: see specific information
   c. Evaluation: base on decrease in parkinsonian symptoms without severe side effects
7. Patient teaching: see specific information

B. Dopaminergic agonists: specific information

1. Mechanism of action
   a. Restore dopamine levels (levodopa, levodopa/carbidopa)
   b. Potentiate the release of dopamine (amantadine)
   c. Activate dopamine receptor sites (bromocriptine)
2. Indications
   a. Levodopa, levodopa-carbidopa: Parkinson's disease
   b. Amantadine: antiviral also used for influenza A prophylaxis and treatment
   c. Bromocriptine: drug also used to treat hyperprolactinemia and experimentally in cocaine abuse
3. Side effects
   a. Levodopa, levodopa/carbidopa: nausea, vomiting, orthostatic hypotension, involuntary body movements
   b. Amantadine: dizziness, confusion, mood changes
   c. Bromocriptine: confusion, involuntary body movements
4. Interactions: pyridoxine (vitamin B_6) inhibits the effects of levodopa
5. Patient teaching
   a. Tell patient on levodopa to avoid excessive vitamin B_6 intake
   b. Advise patient to change positions slowly to minimize the hypotensive effects of levodopa and bromocriptine
6. Drug examples
   a. Levodopa (L-Dopa, Dopar)
   b. Levodopa/carbidopa (Sinemet)
   c. Amantadine (Symmetrel)
   d. Bromocriptine (Parlodel)

C. Anticholinergics: specific information

1. Mechanism of action: decrease cholinergic activity
2. Side effects: blurred vision, dry mouth, constipation, urinary retention
3. Interactions: additive cholinergic effects with other similar-acting drugs
4. Nursing implications: assess bowel and urinary functions for side effects
5. Patient teaching
   a. Warn patient not to take over-the-counter drugs with this medication without consulting physician or pharmacist
   b. Discuss ways to minimize dry mouth and constipation, if problematic
6. Drug examples
   a. Benztropine (Cogentin)
   b. Trihexylphenidyl (Artane)

Points to Remember

Antiparkinsonian drugs do not cure the disease but decrease the symptoms by restoring the balance between the neurotransmitters dopamine and acetylcholine.

Nursing assessment includes monitoring the patient for symptoms of parkinsonism, including rigidity, tremors, akinesia, or bradykinesia.

Besides its use in Parkinson's disease, amantadine is an antiviral used to prevent and treat influenza A.

Besides its use in Parkinson's disease, bromocriptine is used to treat hyperprolactinemia.

Glossary

Akinesia—complete or partial loss of movement

Dopamine—catecholamine involved in the synthesis of norepinephrine

Neurotransmitter—a substance, such as norepinephrine, acetylcholine, or dopamine, that is released when the axon terminal of a presynaptic neuron is excited. The substance then travels across the synapse to the target cell to inhibit or excite it

Parkinson's disease—neurologic disorder characterized by tremors, muscle rigidity and weakness, hypokinesia, and peculiar gait

The Patient with Myasthenia Gravis

Learning Objectives

After studying this section, the reader should be able to:

- Explain the pathophysiology of myasthenia gravis and how it relates to the drugs used to treat this disorder.

- Develop a plan to evaluate the patient with myasthenia gravis for the effectiveness of the medication regimen.

- Explain the importance of compliance with antimyasthenic agents.

- Differentiate between a cholinergic and a myasthenic crisis and discuss the cause and treatment of each.

- Discuss appropriate patient teaching for the patient with myasthenia gravis.

VIII. The Patient with Myasthenia Gravis

A. Antimyasthenic agents: general information

1. Mechanism of action: anticholinesterase drugs relieve the muscle weakness of myasthenia gravis by blocking the breakdown of acetylcholine at the neuromuscular junction
2. Indications: to diagnose or treat myasthenia gravis
3. Contraindications: hypersensitivity
4. Side effects: caused by cholinergic overstimulation
   a. Abdominal pain, nausea, vomiting, diarrhea
   b. Increased salivation and bronchial secretions
   c. Miosis
   d. Sweating
5. Interactions
   a. Additive cholinergic effects with similar-acting drugs
   b. Increase in myasthenic symptoms and hypertension with ganglionic blocking agents (for example, guanethidine)
6. Nursing implications
   a. Assessment: assess neuromuscular status. Monitor patient for signs and symptoms of overdose (cholinergic crisis) and underdose (possible myasthenic crisis)
   b. Implementation: atropine is the antidote for overdose
   c. Evaluation: base on improvement of neuromuscular symptoms or strength without cholinergic symptoms
7. Patient teaching
   a. Explain that therapy is lifelong
   b. Emphasize the importance of taking doses on a specific schedule
   c. Urge patient to carry identification explaining disease and medication regimen

B. Antimyasthenics: specific information

1. Indications
   a. Control of myasthenic symptoms (neostigmine, pyridostigmine)
   b. Diagnosis of disorder and differentiation of cholinergic from myasthenic crisis (edrophonium)
2. Nursing implications
   a. Parenteral doses of neostigmine and pyridostigmine should be much smaller than oral doses because of increased absorption
   b. Edrophonium is given in a 1-ml dose via a tuberculin syringe by a physician
3. Drug examples
   a. Neostigmine (Prostigmin)
   b. Pyridostigmine (Mestinon)
   c. Edrophonium (Tensilon)

Points to Remember

Atropine is the antidote for an overdose of an antimyasthenic agent.

The patient with myasthenia gravis should be informed that therapy will be lifelong.

Nursing assessment includes monitoring the patient with myasthenia gravis for the signs and symptoms of overdose (cholinergic crisis) or underdose (possible myasthenic crisis).

Antimyasthenic medications must be given on time to prevent profuse weakness. This weakness may impede the patient's ability to swallow the drug and may inhibit his ability to breathe.

Glossary

Acetylcholinesterase—an enzyme that stops the action of acetylcholine

Cholinergic crisis—a situation caused by an overdose of an antimyasthenic drug, resulting in muscle weakness, dyspnea, and dysphagia, usually within 1 hour of the drug's administration. Additional symptoms may include increased respiratory secretions and saliva, nausea, vomiting, cramping, diarrhea, and diaphoresis

Myasthenia gravis—disease characterized by muscle weakness that may involve all skeletal muscle groups, including the muscles responsible for swallowing and breathing

Myasthenic crisis—a situation caused by an underdose of or resistance to an antimyasthenic agent. Symptoms include muscle weakness, dyspnea, and dysphagia, and usually occur 3 or more hours after the drug's administration

The Patient Requiring a Sedative/Hypnotic

Learning Objectives

After studying this section, the reader should be able to:

- Explain the mechanism of action for drugs classified as sedatives/hypnotics.

- Describe precautions necessary when administering sedatives/hypnotics.

- Identify the nursing implications during assessment, implementation, and evaluation of the patient receiving sedatives/hypnotics.

- Discuss appropriate patient teaching for the patient receiving sedatives/hypnotics.

- Identify medications commonly used as sedatives/hypnotics.

IX. The Patient Requiring a Sedative/Hypnotic

A. Sedatives/hypnotics: general information

1. Mechanism of action: cause generalized central nervous system (CNS) depression. Many are controlled substances
2. Indications
   a. Anxiety
   b. Insomnia
3. Contraindications and precautions
   a. Do not use in patients with preexisting CNS depression or uncontrolled pain
   b. Do not use during pregnancy
   c. Use with caution in suicidal patients or those previously addicted to drugs
   d. Decrease dosages in elderly patients
4. Side effects: drowsiness
5. Interactions: potentiate CNS depression with alcohol, antihistamines, antidepressants, or phenothiazines
6. Nursing implications
   a. Assessment: assess anxiety or sleep patterns
   b. Implementation: limit amount of medication available to patient. With chronic use, may produce tolerance, and physical and psychological dependence
   c. Evaluation: base on a decrease in anxiety without excessive sedation, or an improvement in sleep patterns
7. Patient teaching
   a. Explain that medication should be decreased gradually following long-term use to prevent withdrawal symptoms
   b. Caution patient to avoid activities requiring alertness until effects of drug are known
   c. Warn patient to avoid alcohol and other CNS depressants while taking these medications

B. Barbiturates: specific information

1. Indications
   a. Rapid-acting: anesthesia (see Section IV)
   b. Short-acting: insomnia, adjunct to anesthesia
   c. Long-acting: insomnia, epilepsy (see Section VI)
2. Side effects: hangover feeling and slurred speech
3. Interactions: increase metabolism and decrease effectiveness of coumadin and oral contraceptives
4. Nursing implications
   a. Assessment: monitor sleep patterns. Barbiturates reduce rapid eye movement (REM) sleep
   b. Implementation: administer I.V. doses slowly; rapid administration may cause respiratory and cardiac depression

    c. Evaluation: base on decreased insomnia without excessive daytime sedation

5. Drug examples
    a. Rapid-acting: thiopenthal sodium (Pentothal)
    b. Short-acting: pentobarbital (Nembutal) and secobarbital (Seconal)
    c. Long-acting: phenobarbital (Luminal)

C. Benzodiazepines: specific information

1. Indications
    a. Anxiety: alprazolam, chlordiazepoxide, diazepam, lorazepam, oxazepam
    b. Alcohol withdrawal: chlordiazepoxide, diazepam, oxazepam
    c. Sedation and amnesia: diazepam, midazolam
    d. Insomnia: flurazepam, temazepam, triazolam
    e. Seizures: clonazepam, diazepam (see Section VI)
    f. Skeletal muscle relaxation: diazepam (see Section XXXIII)

2. Nursing implications: administer I.V. doses slowly to prevent respiratory depression

3. Patient teaching: explain that if dose loses effectiveness after a few weeks, the patient should consult physician, and not increase dose on his own

4. Drug examples
    a. Alprazolam (Xanax)
    b. Chlordiazepoxide (Librium)
    c. Clonazepam (Klonopin)
    d. Diazepam (Valium)
    e. Flurazepam (Dalmane)
    f. Lorazepam (Ativan)
    g. Midazolam (Versed)
    h. Oxazepam (Serax)
    i. Temazepam (Restoril)
    j. Triazolam (Halcion)

D. Other non-barbiturate sedatives/hypnotics: specific information

1. Indications
    a. Anxiety: hydroxyzine, meprobamate, diphenhydramine
    b. Sedation: hydroxyzine, promethazine
    c. Insomnia: chloral hydrate

2. Nursing implications: administer hydroxyzine I.M. via Z-track technique to prevent tissue irritation

3. Drug examples
    a. Chloral hydrate (Noctec, Somnos)
    b. Diphenhydramine (Benadryl): available as an over-the-counter preparation
    c. Hydroxyzine (Atarax, Vistaril)
    d. Meprobamate (Equanil, Miltown)
    e. Promethazine (Phenergan)

Points to Remember

Sedatives/hypnotics are used to treat anxiety and insomnia and as an adjunct to anesthesia.

The actions of sedatives/hypnotics are potentiated by alcohol and other CNS depressants. This effect may be lethal.

Nursing assessment should focus on the patient's anxiety level and his sleep patterns.

These drugs may produce tolerance and physical and psychological dependence. Assess the patient for suicidal tendencies, and limit the amount of medication available to the patient.

Glossary

Hypnotic—a medication that induces sleep or dulls the senses

Insomnia—the inability to sleep, sleep interrupted by periods of wakefulness, or sleep that ends prematurely

Sedative—a medication that exerts a soothing or tranquilizing effect

Withdrawal symptoms—barbiturate withdrawal is characterized by anxiety, restlessness, tremors, weakness, dizziness, nausea, vomiting, nightmares, hallucinations, and seizures. Withdrawal from benzodiazepine therapy is characterized by sleep disturbances, irritability, nervousness, abdominal and muscle cramps, confusion, nausea, vomiting, sweating, and seizures. Withdrawal symptoms usually occur after prolonged high-dose therapy

The Patient with a Psychotic Disorder

Learning Objectives

After studying this section, the reader should be able to:

- Explain the rationale for the use of antipsychotics.

- List the indications for antipsychotic drugs.

- Identify the nursing implications during assessment, implementation, and evaluation of the patient receiving antipsychotic drugs.

- Discuss appropriate patient teaching for the patient receiving antipsychotic drugs.

X. The Patient with a Psychotic Disorder

A. Antipsychotics: general information

1. Mechanism of action: block the neurotransmitter, dopamine, in the limbic system of the brain, inhibiting the transmission of the neural impulse. As antiemetics, they inhibit the medullary chemoreceptor trigger zone
2. Indications
   a. Acute and chronic psychoses
   b. Nausea and vomiting: chlorpromazine, prochlorperazine
   c. Anesthesia: droperidol (in combination with fentanyl)
3. Contraindications and precautions
   a. Do not use in patients with narrow-angle glaucoma
   b. Do not use in patients with central nervous system (CNS) depression
   c. Withhold 48 hours before and 24 hours after metrizamide myelography because these drugs may lower seizure threshold
4. Side effects
   a. Extrapyramidal reactions
   b. Tardive dyskinesia
   c. Sedation
   d. Anticholinergic effects: include dry mouth, blurred vision, constipation
   e. Photosensitivity: may cause temporary blue-gray skin pigmentation on exposed surfaces
   f. Heat intolerance: antipsychotics impair body temperature regulation
5. Interactions
   a. Antipsychotics potentiate alcohol and CNS depressants
   b. Additive hypotension occurs with antihypertensives and nitrates
   c. Antacids decrease absorption
6. Nursing implications
   a. Assessment: assess mental status and monitor for extrapyramidal symptoms. Assess nausea and vomiting when used as an antiemetic
   b. Implementation: decrease doses of narcotic analgesics to one quarter to one third of the normal dose for 8 hours following the administration of droperidol/fentanyl (Innovar). Monitor for orthostatic hypotension following parenteral doses
   c. Evaluation: base on improved ability to interact with others and participate in activities of daily living. Evaluate for resolution of nausea and vomiting when used an antiemetic
7. Patient teaching
   a. Emphasize the importance of compliance with therapy; drug may not produce desired effect for several weeks. Withdrawal should be gradual
   b. Warn against taking alcohol or other CNS depressants with these drugs
   c. Discuss ways to minimize dry mouth and constipation
   d. Recommend use of sunscreen and protective clothing, and urge patient to avoid extremes of temperature

e. Caution patient to avoid driving and activities requiring alertness until effects of drug are known

f. Alert patient not to take antacids within 1 hour of these medications

B. Phenothiazines: specific information
1. Indications
   a. Antipsychotic: chlorpromazine, fluphenazine, prochlorperazine, promazine, thioridazine, trifluoperazine
   b. Antiemetic: chlorpromazine, prochlorperazine
2. Drug examples
   a. Chlorpromazine (Thorazine)
   b. Fluphenazine (Prolixin)
   c. Prochlorperazine (Compazine)
   d. Promazine (Sparine)
   e. Thioridazine (Mellaril)
   f. Trifluoperazine (Stelazine)

C. Butyrophenones: specific information
1. Indications
   a. Antipsychotic: haloperidol
   b. Tourette's syndrome: haloperidol
   c. Antiemetic: droperidol
   d. Adjunct to anesthesia: droperidol
2. Drug examples
   a. Haloperidol (Haldol)
   b. Droperidol (Inapsine)

Points to Remember

Antipsychotic agents are used as adjunctive therapy for psychoses and for nausea and vomiting.

The nurse needs to assess the mental status of the patient taking antipsychotic agents. Loss of contact with reality may mean noncompliance.

The potential for suicide should also be assessed and a limited amount of drugs given to the patient at risk.

Nursing assessment of the patient taking phenothiazines includes monitoring for the signs and symptoms of tardive dyskinesia, which may be irreversible.

Glossary

Extrapyramidal symptoms—movements caused by an imbalance in the extrapyramidal system of the brain and characterized by pill-rolling motions, drooling, tremors, rigidity, and shuffling gait

Psychosis—major mental illness characterized by personality disintegration and loss of touch with reality; often includes hallucinations and delusions

Tardive dyskinesia—a late-developing, drug-induced, potentially irreversible movement disorder characterized by involuntary movements of the face, mouth, tongue, jaw, and extremities

Tourette's syndrome—neurologic disorder characterized by multiple tics (blinking, grimacing, shrugging) that progresses to grunting, shouting, barking, and, often, compulsive swearing

The Patient with an Affective Disorder

Learning Objectives

After studying this section, the reader should be able to:

- Describe the mechanism of action of the antidepressant and antimanic drugs.

- List the indications for antidepressant and antimanic drugs.

- Name the common side effects of antidepressant and antimanic drugs.

- Identify the nursing implications during assessment, implementation, and evaluation of the patient receiving antidepressant and antimanic drugs.

- Discuss appropriate patient teaching for the patient receiving antidepressant and antimanic drugs.

XI. The Patient with an Affective Disorder

A. Antidepressants/antimanic agents: general information

1. Mechanism of action: impair the inactivation of norepinephrine and/or serotonin, prolonging their presence within the central nervous system (CNS) synapses
2. Indications
   a. Treatment of depression (antidepressants, monoamine oxidase [MAO] inhibitors)
   b. Treatment of bipolar affective disorders (lithium)
3. Contraindications
   a. Narrow-angle glaucoma (antidepressants)
   b. Pregnancy (antidepressants, MAO inhibitors, lithium)
4. Side effects: see specific information
5. Interactions: see specific information
6. Nursing implications
   a. Assessment: assess mental status for mood changes or suicidal tendencies
   b. Implementation: see specific information
   c. Evaluation: base on decreased anxiety, increased appetite, improved energy level, and improved sleep in patients on antidepressant therapy. Effectiveness of lithium is based on resolution of symptoms of mania and decreased mood swings in bipolar disorders
7. Patient teaching: see specific information

B. Antidepressants: specific information

1. Indications
   a. Depression
   b. Enuresis: imipramine
   c. Anxiety: doxepin
   d. Neurogenic pain (investigational): amitriptyline, doxepin, imipramine
2. Contraindications and precautions: may lower seizure threshold. Discontinue 48 hours before and 24 hours after metrizamide myelography
3. Side effects
   a. Orthostatic hypotension, tachycardia
   b. Blurred vision, dry mouth, constipation
   c. Drowsiness, sedation, lethargy, fatigue
4. Interactions
   a. Will produce additive CNS depression with alcohol, antihistamines, and other CNS depressants
   b. May decrease effectiveness of antihypertensives
   c. May cause hypertensive crisis when used with MAO inhibitors
5. Patient teaching
   a. Inform patient of importance of compliance with therapy; drug may not produce noticeable effect for 2 weeks or more. Antidepressants should be discontinued gradually

      b. Warn patient to avoid alcohol and over-the-counter drugs
      c. Caution patient to avoid driving or other activities requiring alertness
         until effects of drug are known
  6. Drug examples
      a. Amitriptyline (Elavil, Endep)
      b. Doxepin (Adapin, Sinequan)
      c. Imipramine (Tofranil)
      d. Maprotiline (Ludiomil)
      e. Trazodone (Desyrel)

C. Monoamine oxidase (MAO) inhibitors: specific information
  1. Indications: used in treatment of depression in patients who do not tolerate
     other forms of therapy
  2. Side effects
      a. Restlessness, insomnia, dizziness, headache
      b. Orthostatic hypotension, hypertensive crisis
      c. Constipation, dry mouth, nausea, vomiting
  3. Interactions
      a. Hypertensive crisis may occur with tyramine-containing foods,
         amphetamines, methyldopa, levodopa, dopamine, epinephrine,
         norepinephrine, antidepressants, guanethidine, reserpine,
         vasoconstrictors, and nasal decongestants
      b. Hypertension, hypotension, coma, or convulsions may occur with
         narcotic analgesics. Should be discontinued several weeks before
         surgery
  4. Nursing implications: do not administer in the evening; may cause insomnia
  5. Patient teaching
      a. Emphasize the importance of compliance; drug effects may not
         be noticeable for 1 to 4 weeks. Should be discontinued gradually
      b. Caution patient to avoid alcohol and foods containing tyramine
      c. Instruct patient to carry identification describing disease and
         drug regimen
  6. Drug examples
      a. Isocarboxazid (Marplan)
      b. Phenelzine (Nardil)
      c. Tranylcypromine (Parnate)

D. Antimanic agents: specific information
  1. Side effects
      a. Tremors, headache, impaired memory, lethargy, fatigue
      b. Nausea, anorexia, abdominal pain
  2. Interactions
      a. Diuretics, methyldopa, probenecid, and nonsterodial anti-inflammatory
         agents may increase risk of toxicity
      b. Aminophylline, phenothiazine, sodium bicarbonate, and increased
         sodium intake may increase renal excretion and decrease effectiveness

3. Nursing implications
   a. Monitor lithium levels and assess patient for signs and symptoms of toxicity
   b. Administer with food to minimize GI irritation
4. Patient teaching
   a. Instruct patient to drink 2 to 3 liters of fluid daily; eat a high-sodium diet; avoid excessive amounts of coffee, tea, and cola (which have a diuretic effect); and avoid activities that cause excess sodium loss because low sodium levels predispose patient to toxicity
   b. Warn patient to consult physician or pharmacist before taking over-the-counter drugs
5. Drug examples
   a. Lithium carbonate (Eskalith, Lithane, Lithonate)
   b. Lithium citrate (Cibalith-S)

Points to Remember

Antidepressants and monoamine oxidase inhibitors are used to treat depression.

The patient taking drugs for an affective disorder should be assessed for suicidal tendencies.

Ingestion of foods containing tyramine (red wine, beer, aged cheeses, yeast, avocados, bananas, yogurt, smoked or pickled fish, chocolate, overripe fruit, caffeine-containing beverages) by the patient taking monoamine oxidase inhibitors may cause a hypertensive crisis.

Lithium toxicity, manifested by vomiting, diarrhea, slurred speech, decreased coordination, drowsiness, muscle weakness, and twitching, may be precipitated by decreased sodium levels.

Glossary

Bipolar affective disorder—affective disorder characterized by periods of mania and overactivity and/or periods of depression and decreased activity, or by alternation of the two

Enuresis—involuntary urination, usually referred to as nocturnal enuresis (bed-wetting)

Norepinephrine—adrenergic hormone that increases blood pressure by vasoconstriction without affecting heart output

Serotonin—neurotransmitter; a powerful vasoconstrictor; thought to be involved in sleep and sensory perception

The Patient Requiring a Cardiac Glycoside

Learning Objectives

After studing this section, the reader should be able to:

- Describe the general mechanisms of action of cardiac glycosides.

- Identify the nursing implications during assessment, implementation, and evaluation of the patient receiving cardiac glycosides.

- Discuss appropriate patient teaching for the patient receiving cardiac glycosides.

- Relate the additional nursing implications pertinent to the administration of this medication to the geriatric patient.

XII. The Patient Requiring a Cardiac Glycoside

A. **Cardiac glycosides: general information**
   1. Mechanism of action
       a. Positive inotrope: increases force of contraction
       b. Negative chronotrope: depresses sinoatrial (SA) node and decreases velocity through atrioventricular (AV) node; slows heart rate
   2. Indications
       a. Congestive heart failure (often with diuretics)
       b. Control of ventricular rate in atrial tachyarrhythmias (fibrillation, flutter, paroxysmal atrial tachycardia)
   3. Contraindications and precautions
       a. Cardiac glycosides are contraindicated in uncontrolled ventricular dysrhythmias, idiopathic hypertrophic subaortic stenosis, constrictive pericarditis, and complete heart block
       b. Hypokalemia, hypercalcemia, hypomagnesemia, and hypothyroidism increase the risk of toxicity
       c. Cardiac glycosides should be used with caution in patients with acute myocardial infarction
       d. Elderly patients may be more sensitive to toxic effects
   4. Side effects
       a. Side effects include nausea, vomiting, diarrhea, fatigue, weakness, bradycardia
       b. Toxic effects are characterized by anorexia, nausea, vomiting, visual disturbances, confusion, bradycardia, heart block, premature ventricular contractions, and tachyarrhythmias
   5. Interactions
       a. Potassium-wasting diuretics and other drugs causing potassium loss may increase the risk of toxicity
       b. Quinidine, verapamil, and nifedipine increase digoxin levels and may lead to toxicity
       c. Additive bradycardia occurs with beta-adrenergic blocking agents
       d. Antacids decrease absorption
   6. Nursing implications
       a. Assessment: monitor apical pulse, digoxin and electrolyte levels, and renal function before administering. Assess for signs and symptoms of toxicity, especially in the elderly and during digitalization. Digoxin Immune Fab (Digibind) is the antidote
       b. Implementation: do not alternate dosage forms; bioavailability of capsules is not equal to that of tablets or elixir
       c. Evaluation: base on a decrease in severity of congestive heart failure or atrial dysrhythmias and an increase in cardiac output
   7. Patient teaching
       a. Explain how to take this medication. Warn against doubling up on missed doses. Advise patient to consult physician before discontinuing

b. Instruct patient on correct method for monitoring pulse before taking drug. Notify physician if pulse rate is less than 60 beats/minute or more than 100 beats/minute

c. Advise patient of the signs and symptoms of digitalis toxicity and congestive heart failure

B. Digitalis glycosides: specific information
1. Nursing implications
   a. Digoxin is metabolized and excreted by the kidneys; dose must be reduced in renal impairment
   b. Digitoxin is metabolized by the liver and excreted by the kidneys; used more commonly for patients in renal failure
2. Drug examples
   a. Digoxin (Lanoxin, Lanoxicaps)
   b. Digitoxin (Crystodigin, Purodigin)

Points to Remember

The majority of cardiac glycosides are digitalis glycosides, including digoxin and digitoxin.

Patients taking digitalis glycosides must be continually monitored for toxicity.

Hypokalemia places the patient taking a digitalis glycoside at increased risk for toxicity.

Dosage forms of cardiac glycosides should not be alternated because the bioavailability of capsules is not equal to that of tablets or elixir.

Glossary

Atrial fibrillation—extremely rapid atrial contraction (200 to 400 contractions a minute) with a variable ventricular contraction response

Bioavailability—rate and extent to which a drug enters the circulation, thus gaining access to the target tissue

Digitalization—administration of a larger-than-maintenance dose (loading dose) of digitalis to attain a therapeutic blood level rapidly. The patient must be closely observed for toxicity

Idiopathic—of unknown cause

The Patient with Dysrhythmias

Learning Objectives

After studying this section, the reader should be able to:

- Describe the mechanism of action of antiarrhythmics.

- Name the common side effects of antiarrhythmics.

- Identify the nursing implications during assessment, implementation, and evaluation of the patient receiving antiarrhythmics.

- Discuss appropriate patient teaching for the patient receiving antiarrhythmics.

XIII. The Patient with Dysrhythmias

A. Antiarrhythmics: general information

1. Mechanism of action: correct cardiac dysrhythmias; classified by effects on cardiac conduction tissue
2. Indications: cardiac dysrhythmias
3. Contraindications: see specific information
4. Side effects: see specific information
5. Interactions: see specific information
6. Nursing implications
    a. Assessment: assess vital signs and monitor EKG
    b. Implementation: administer antiarrhythmics around the clock. I.V. infusions must be on infusion pumps for accuracy
    c. Evaluation: base on the suppression of dysrhythmias without side effects
7. Patient teaching
    a. Explain the purpose of these drugs and the need to comply with the therapeutic regimen
    b. Instruct patient to monitor his pulse daily

B. Type I antiarrhythmics: specific information

1. Mechanism of action
    a. Increase the threshold of excitability
    b. Prolong the refractory period and inhibit reentry
2. Indications
    a. Atrial fibrillation
    b. Premature ventricular contractions
    c. Ventricular tachycardia
3. Contraindications and precautions
    a. Contraindicated in atrioventricular (AV) block and in patients allergic to amide-type local anesthetics
    b. Use cautiously in patients with congestive heart failure
4. Side effects
    a. Nausea and GI distress
    b. Hypotension, heart failure, heart block
5. Interactions
    a. Additive hypotension occurs with antihypertensives
    b. Cimetidine increases blood levels of disopyramide and lidocaine
    c. Risk of digitalis glycoside toxicity increases when given with digoxin or digitoxin
6. Nursing implications: never administer lidocaine I.V. containing epinephrine or preservatives to treat dysrhythmias
7. Drug examples
    a. Disopyramide (Norpace)
    b. Flecainide (Tambocor)
    c. Mexilitine (Mexitil)

    d. Lidocaine (Xylocaine)
    e. Phenytoin (Dilantin)
    f. Procainamide (Pronestyl, Procan)
    g. Quinidine (Quinidex, Quinora, Quinaglute)
    h. Tocainide (Tonocard)

C. Type II antiarrhythmics (see Section II, beta-adrenergic blocking agents): specific information
  1. Mechanism of action: decrease sympathetic activity at the sinoatrial (SA) and AV nodes, decreasing automaticity and increasing the refractory period
  2. Indications
    a. Sinus tachycardia
    b. Atrial fibrillation and flutter
    c. Ventricular dysrhythmias (propranolol)
  3. Contraindications and precautions: contraindicated in heart block, congestive heart failure, sinus bradycardia, asthma, valvular disease
  4. Side effects
    a. Hypotension, congestive heart failure, bronchospasm, bradycardia, dysrhythmias, heart block
    b. Fatigue, dizziness, GI distress
  5. Interactions: diuretics, phenothiazines, and calcium channel blockers increase hypotensive effects
  6. Patient teaching
    a. Advise patient to monitor for weight gain
    b. Inform patient that medications should be discontinued gradually under physician's supervision
  7. Drug examples
    a. Acebutolol (Sectral)
    b. Propranolol (Inderal)

D. Type III antiarrhythmics: specific information
  1. Mechanism of action: prolong the duration of the action potential and lengthen the absolute refractory period
  2. Indications
    a. Ventricular dysrhythmias
    b. Ventricular tachycardia and fibrillation
  3. Side effects
    a. Hypotension (bretylium), congestive heart failure, bradycardia (amiodarone)
    b. Nausea and vomiting
    c. Photosensitivity: bluish discoloration of skin, corneal microdeposits (amiodarone)
    d. Hypothyroidism, peripheral neuropathy, tremor, poor coordination, abnormal gait (amiodarone)
  4. Interactions
    a. Use with digitalis may increase dysrhythmias
    b. Use with quinidine and procainamide may increase hypotension

5. Nursing implications
   a. Assessment: assess lung, thyroid, and neurologic functions of patient taking amiodarone
   b. Implementation: keep patient supine and monitor blood pressure for hypotension after administering bretylium
6. Patient teaching
   a. Instruct patient on bretylium to change positions slowly to minimize orthostatic hypotension
   b. Advise patient taking amiodarone to use sunscreen and protective clothing to prevent photosensitivity reactions
7. Drug examples
   a. Bretylium (Bretylol)
   b. Amiodarone (Cordarone)

E. Type IV antiarrhythmics: specific information
1. Mechanism of action: block the slow inward calcium channel, slowing conduction through the AV node
2. Indications
   a. Atrial fibrillation or flutter
   b. Supraventricular tachycardias
3. Contraindications and precautions: use cautiously in AV block, severe congestive heart failure, and sick sinus syndrome
4. Side effects
   a. Hypotension, bradycardia, edema
   b. Dizziness, constipation
5. Interactions
   a. Type IV antiarrhythmics increase risk of digitalis toxicity
   b. Beta-adrenergic blocking agents may cause increased risk of bradycardia and congestive heart failure
   c. Additive hypotension occurs with antihypertensives and nitrates
6. Patient teaching: advise patient to change positions slowly to minimize orthostatic hypotension
7. Drug example: verapamil (Calan, Isoptin)

Points to Remember

Antiarrhythmics suppress selected dysrhythmias by inhibiting abnormal pathways of electrical conduction through the heart. Patients must be monitored closely because these drugs may create new dysrhythmias.

Intravenous forms of the antiarrhythmic drugs are very potent and require an infusion pump to ensure accurate administration.

The patient taking an antiarrhythmic should monitor his pulse daily.

When lidocaine is used to treat dysrhythmias, it should never be used in an I.V. solution containing epinephrine or preservatives.

Glossary

Action potential—electrical impulse across nerve or muscle fibers when they have been stimulated

Atrioventricular (AV) block—slowed conduction or cessation of heart's excitatory impulse, occurring at AV node, bundle of His, or its branches

Refractory period—period of relaxation following muscle excitement

Sick sinus syndrome—degeneration of conductive tissue that maintains heart rhythm

The Patient with Hypertension

Learning Objectives
After studying this section, the reader should be able to:

- Describe the mechanism of action and the rationale for use of the various antihypertensive agents.

- Name the common side effects of antihypertensive agents.

- Identify the nursing implications during assessment, implementation, and evaluation of the patient receiving antihypertensive agents.

- Discuss appropriate patient teaching for the patient receiving antihypertensive agents.

XIV. The Patient with Hypertension

A. Antihypertensives: general information
1. Mechanism of action: mechanisms of lowering blood pressure are classified according to site of action
2. Indications: hypertension
3. Contraindications and precautions: see specific information
4. Side effects: see specific information
5. Interactions
    a. Additive hypotension occurs with similar-acting drugs and alcohol
    b. Antihistamines, nonsteroidal anti-inflammatory agents, sympathomimetic bronchodilators, decongestants, appetite suppressants, and antidepressants decrease effectiveness
6. Nursing implications
    a. Assessment: monitor vital signs and assess for other risk factors of hypertension. Clonidine, methyldopa, and reserpine may increase depression in patients with a history of mental depression; monitor closely
    b. Implementation: administer I.V. infusions via infusion pump for accuracy
    c. Evaluation: base on decrease in blood pressure without serious side effects
7. Patient teaching
    a. Instruct patient to monitor blood pressure weekly
    b. Explain the importance of compliance with therapy. Do not double up on missed doses. Rebound hypertension may occur if drugs are stopped abruptly
    c. Advise patient to change positions slowly to minimize orthostatic hypotension. Caution against hot baths or showers
    d. Advise patient to monitor for weight gain and fluid retention
    e. Warn against excessive amounts of coffee, tea, cola, or alcohol
    f. Encourage patient to comply with additional interventions: weight reduction, low-sodium diet, smoking cessation, regular exercise, stress management
    g. Tell patient to notify physician if side effects are intolerable

B. Centrally acting adrenergic inhibitors: specific information
1. Mechanism of action: reduce sympathetic outflow from the central nervous system (CNS), causing peripheral vasodilation. Often combined with a diuretic
2. Side effects
    a. Drowsiness, dry mouth, edema, impotence, depression
    b. Constipation, dizziness (clonidine)
    c. Headache, paresthesias, sleep disturbances (methyldopa)
3. Patient teaching
    a. Explain that clonidine is best taken at bedtime
    b. Instruct patient in the use of transdermal clonidine

4. Drug examples
   a. Clonidine (Catapres, Catapres TTS)
   b. Methyldopa (Aldomet)

C. Peripherally acting adrenergic inhibitors: specific information
   1. Mechanism of action: reduce the effects of norepinephrine at the peripheral nerve endings. Often combined with a diuretic
   2. Side effects
      a. Edema, diarrhea, nasal stuffiness, orthostatic hypotension
      b. Drowsiness, depression, GI irritation, impotence (reserpine)
      c. Weakness, ejaculation failure, bradycardia (guanethidine)
   3. Drug examples
      a. Reserpine (Serpasil)
      b. Guanethidine (Ismelin)

D. Peripheral vasodilators: specific information
   1. Mechanism of action: act directly on the arteries alone, or both arteries and veins to decrease peripheral vascular resistance. Often combined with beta-adrenergic blockers
   2. Indications
      a. Hypertension (hydralazine, minoxidil, prazosin)
      b. Hypertensive crisis (diazoxide, sodium nitroprusside)
   3. Side effects: fluid retention, tachycardia, orthostatic hypotension, nausea, severe hypotension with I.V. doses
   4. Drug examples
      a. Hydralazine (Apresoline)
      b. Minoxidil (Loniten)
      c. Prazosin (Minipress)
      d. Diazoxide (Hyperstat)
      e. Sodium nitroprusside (Nipride)

E. Beta-adrenergic blocking agents (see Section II): specific information
   1. Mechanism of action: compete with epinephrine for beta-adrenergic receptor sites; inhibit response to beta-adrenergic stimuli
   2. Contraindications and precautions: contraindicated in congestive heart failure, bradycardia, and asthma
   3. Side effects: bradycardia, nausea, vomiting, fatigue, orthostatic hypotension
   4. Patient teaching: explain that these drugs should be discontinued gradually
   5. Drug examples
      a. Acebutolol (Sectral)
      b. Atenolol (Tenormin)
      c. Labetalol (Normodyne, Trandate)
      d. Metoprolol (Lopressor)
      e. Nadolol (Corgard)
      f. Propranolol (Inderal)

F. Angiotensin antagonists: specific information
1. Mechanism of action: block conversion of angiotensin I to II, preventing peripheral vasoconstriction
2. Side effects: proteinuria, rash, tachycardia, palpitations, dizziness, lightheadedness, fainting
3. Drug examples
   a. Captopril (Capoten)
   b. Enalapril (Vasotec)

G. Calcium channel blockers: specific information
1. Mechanism of action: block the slow channel, preventing calcium from entering the cell; this causes vasodilation
2. Side effects: edema, flushing, dizziness, headache, nausea
3. Nursing implications: nifedipine may be given sublingually; puncture end of capsule and squeeze liquid under the tongue
4. Drug examples
   a. Nifedipine (Procardia)
   b. Diltiazem (Cardizem)
   c. Verapamil (Calan, Isoptin)

H. Diuretics (see Section XVI): specific information
1. Mechanism of action: inhibit sodium and chloride reabsorption, causing increased urine output and decreased edema
2. Side effects: hypokalemia, hyperglycemia, skin rash, orthostatic hypotension, fatigue, dizziness
3. Drug examples
   a. Chlorothiazide (Diuril)
   b. Chlorthalidone (Hygroton)
   c. Furosemide (Lasix)
   d. Hydrochlorothiazide (HydroDIURIL)

Points to Remember

The patient with a history of mental depression should be monitored closely when taking antihypertensives, because some antihypertensives may increase depression.

Clonidine is best taken at bedtime.

Intravenous forms of the antihypertensive drugs are potent and require an infusion pump to ensure accurate administration.

The patient on antihypertensive medications should be taught the importance of compliance with therapy as well as with additional interventions to manage hypertension.

The patient on antihypertensive medications should be taught to change position slowly to avoid orthostatic hypotension.

Glossary

Angiotensin—polypeptide in blood that causes vasoconstriction. Angiotensin I, which is physiologically inactive, is the precursor of angiotensin II

Hypertensive crisis—an emergency situation in which the diastolic blood pressure is usually greater than 120 mm Hg

Paresthesia—abnormal sensations, including numbness, prickling, and tingling, with no known cause

Proteinuria—presence of abnormally large amount of protein, usually albumin, in urine

The Patient Requiring Vasodilating Agents

Learning Objectives

After studying this section, the reader should be able to:

● Describe the mechanism of action of the various vasodilating agents.

● Name the common side effects of vasodilating agents.

● Identify the nursing implications during assessment, implementation, and evaluation of the patient receiving vasodilating agents.

● Discuss appropriate patient teaching for the patient receiving vasodilating agents.

XV. The Patient Requiring Vasodilating Agents

A. Vasodilating agents: general information

1. Mechanism of action: reduce oxygen demand or increase coronary blood supply (see specific information)
2. Indications: angina pectoris
3. Contraindications: uncontrolled hypotension or hypertension
4. Side effects: flushing, headache, hypotension
5. Interactions: additive hypotension with alcohol, beta-adrenergic blocking agents, calcium channel blockers, and antihypertensives
6. Nursing implications
    a. Assessment: assess location, duration, intensity, and precipitating factors of the patient's anginal pain
    b. Evaluation: base on decreased frequency and severity of anginal attacks and increased activity tolerance
7. Patient teaching
    a. Advise patient to change positions slowly to minimize orthostatic hypotension. Caution against hot baths or showers
    b. Warn against use of alcohol with these drugs

B. Nitrates: specific information

1. Mechanism of action: produce vasodilation, decrease preload and afterload, and decrease myocardial oxygen consumption
2. Indications
    a. Acute treatment and prophylactic management of angina
    b. Surgical hypotension (I.V. nitroglycerin)
3. Patient teaching
    a. Instruct patient in correct method of using and storing nitroglycerin sublingual tablets. Explain that for acute anginal attacks, patient should sit down and use drug at first sign of attack. May repeat if no relief in 5 minutes. If no relief after 3 tablets in 15 minutes, go to nearest emergency room
    b. Inform patient that headache is a common side effect and should decrease with continued therapy. May treat with aspirin or acetaminophen
    c. Teach patient how to apply transdermal ointment or patches
4. Drug examples
    a. Nitroglycerin (NTG, Nitro-Bid, Nitrospan, Nitrodisc, Nitro-Dur, Nitrol, Transderm-Nitro)
    b. Isosorbide dinitrate (Isordil, Sorbitrate, Isordil Tembids)

C. Calcium channel blockers (see Section XIV): specific information

1. Mechanism of action: dilate coronary arteries, prevent coronary vasospasm, and dilate peripheral arteries
2. Indications
    a. Stable and unstable angina
    b. Vasospastic (Prinzmetal's) angina

3. Side effects
   a. Reflex increase in heart rate, peripheral edema (nifedipine)
   b. Constipation, dizziness (diltiazem, verapamil)
4. Interactions: nifedipine may increase risk of digitalis toxicity
5. Patient teaching: tell the patient that he may need to continue concurrent nitrate therapy
6. Drug examples
   a. Nifedipine (Procardia)
   b. Diltiazem (Cardiazem)
   c. Verapamil (Calan, Isoptin)

D. Beta-adrenergic blockers (Sections II and XIV): specific information

1. Mechanism of action: decrease myocardial oxygen needs by decreasing heart rate and force of contraction
2. Drug examples
   a. Atenolol (Tenormin)
   b. Metoprolol (Lopressor)
   c. Nadolol (Corgard)
   d. Propranolol (Inderal)

Points to Remember

Vasodilating agents are used to treat angina.

Nitroglycerin is available intravenously and as a sublingual tablet, transdermal ointment, or patch.

Symptoms of angina are similar to those of a myocardial infarction.

Patients on vasodilators should be taught to recognize the difference between the symptoms of angina and of myocardial infarction and to use guidelines on when to seek emergency medical assistance.

Glossary

Afterload—the amount of tension the ventricle must develop to open the semilunar valve and eject the blood

Myocardial oxygen consumption—the amount of oxygen the heart uses during each beat. As the work of the heart increases, as with increased preload and afterload, the myocardial oxygen consumption also increases

Preload—the volume of blood in the ventricles at the end of diastole. Excessive volumes overstretch myocardial fibers, causing decreased cardiac output

Vasospastic (Prinzmetal's) angina—uncommon form of angina in which attacks occur during rest rather than during activity

The Patient Requiring a Diuretic

Learning Objectives

After studying this section, the reader should be able to:

- Identify medications commonly used as diuretics.

- Explain the mechanism of action and rationale for use of thiazide, loop, potassium-sparing, and osmotic diuretics.

- Describe the major side effects of each class of diuretics.

- Identify the nursing implications during assessment, implementation, and evaluation of the patient receiving each class of diuretics.

- Discuss appropriate patient teaching for the patient receiving each class of diuretics.

XVI. The Patient Requiring a Diuretic

A. Diuretics: general information

1. Mechanism of action: see specific information
2. Indications
    a. Hypertension, edema, congestive heart failure (thiazide or loop diuretics)
    b. Conservation of potassium in patients on thiazide or loop diuretics (potassium-sparing diuretics)
    c. Glaucoma (carbonic anhydrase inhibitors, osmotic diuretics)
    d. Cerebral edema (osmotic diuretics)
    e. Hypercalcemia from bone metastases (loop diuretics)
3. Contraindications: pregnancy and lactation (except thiazide diuretics)
4. Side effects: see specific information
5. Interactions: additive hypotension with antihypertensives
6. Nursing implications
    a. Assessment: monitor blood pressure, intake and output, lung sounds, weight, and edema daily. Monitor electrolytes
    b. Implementation: administer diuretics in the morning to prevent disruption of sleep
    c. Evaluation: base on decreased blood pressure, edema, intraocular pressure, or cerebral edema without electrolyte imbalance
7. Patient teaching
    a. Encourage patient to comply with interventions for hypertension (smoking cessation, weight loss, exercise, stress management, low-sodium diet)
    b. Advise patient to change positions slowly to minimize orthostatic hypotension
    c. Warn against alcohol use with these drugs

B. Thiazide diuretics: specific information

1. Mechanism of action: increase excretion of sodium and water by inhibiting sodium reabsorption in the distal tubule
2. Contraindications and precautions: contraindicated with sensitivity to sulfa drugs
3. Side effects
    a. Hypokalemia, hyperglycemia, dysrhythmias, weakness
    b. Orthostatic hypotension, photosensitivity, muscle cramps
4. Interactions
    a. Additive hypokalemia with other potassium-depleting drugs; this may increase risk of digitalis toxicity
    b. Decreased excretion of lithium; may cause toxicity

5. Nursing implications: monitor digoxin levels in patients on concurrent therapy
6. Patient teaching: advise patient to use sunscreen and protective clothing to prevent photosensitivity reactions
7. Drug examples
   a. Chlorothiazide (Diuril)
   b. Hydrochlorothiazide (HydroDIURIL, Esidrix)
   c. Chlorthalidone (Hygroton)

C. Loop diuretics: specific information
1. Mechanism of action: inhibit the reabsorption of sodium and chloride from the loop of Henle and the distal tubule
2. Side effects: metabolic alkalosis, hypovolemia, dehydration, hyponatremia, hypokalemia, hypochloremia, hypomagnesemia
3. Interactions
   a. Additive hypokalemia with other potassium-depleting drugs; this may increase the risk of digitalis toxicity
   b. Decreased excretion of lithium; may cause toxicity
   c. Increased risk of ototoxicity with aminoglycosides
4. Nursing implications: monitor digoxin levels in patients on concurrent therapy
5. Patient teaching: advise patient to use sunscreen and protective clothing to prevent photosensitivity reactions
6. Drug examples
   a. Furosemide (Lasix)
   b. Ethacrynic acid (Edecrin)

D. Potassium-sparing diuretics: specific information
1. Mechanism of action: act at distal tubule, causing excretion of sodium, bicarbonate, and calcium, while conserving potassium
2. Side effects: hyperkalemia, nausea, vomiting, diarrhea
3. Interactions
   a. Captopril, enalapril, or potassium supplements may cause hyperkalemia
   b. These diuretics decrease lithium excretion, which may lead to toxicity
   c. Aspirin may decrease diuretic response
4. Patient teaching: instruct patient to avoid salt substitutes and foods high in potassium unless directed otherwise by physician
5. Drug examples
   a. Spironolactone (Aldactone)
   b. Triamterene (Dyrenium)

E. Osmotic diuretics: specific information
 1. Mechanism of action: increase osmotic pressure of glomerular filtrate, inhibiting reabsorption of water and electrolytes
 2. Side effects: hyponatremia, dehydration, fluid overload from osmotic effects
 3. Nursing implications: monitor vital signs, urine output, and central venous pressure. Assess neurologic status and intracranial pressure
 4. Drug example: mannitol (Osmitrol)

F. Carbonic anhydrase inhibitors: specific information
 1. Mechanism of action: inhibit carbonic anhydrase in the eye, decreasing the secretions of the aqueous humor
 2. Side effects: metabolic acidosis
 3. Drug example: acetazolamide (Diamox)

Points to Remember

Diuretics are drugs that increase the secretion of urine by increasing the glomerular filtration rate or by decreasing reabsorption from the tubules.

The thiazide and loop diuretics, used to treat hypertension, edema, and congestive heart failure, may cause electrolyte imbalances, especially hypokalemia.

Potassium-sparing diuretics are used to conserve potassium in patients taking thiazide or loop diuretics. These patients must be monitored for hyperkalemia.

Osmotic diuretics create an osmotic gradient in the glomerular filtrate and in the blood. In the glomerular filtrate, the gradient prevents the reabsorption of sodium and water. In the blood, the gradient draws fluid from the intracellular spaces into the intravascular space. The increased intravascular volume may cause fluid overload if kidney function is impaired.

Carbonic anhydrase inhibitors are rarely used as diuretics because of the potential for metabolic acidosis, but they are commonly used to treat glaucoma.

Glossary

Distal tubule—the portion of the renal tubule following the loop of Henle that makes the final changes in the urine for regulation of water and acid-base balance

Glomerular filtrate—the fluid remaining in the renal tubule following the filtration of the blood in the glomerulus

Loop of Henle—the descending and ascending loops of the renal tubule that alter urine osmolality by changes in the permeability to water and sodium

Osmotic pressure—the pressure that develops between two solutions of different concentrations that are separated by a semipermeable membrane

Ototoxicity—potentially irreversible damage to the auditory and vestibular branches of the eighth cranial nerve; may result in loss of hearing or loss of balance

The Patient with Anemia

Learning Objectives

After studying this section, the reader should be able to:

- Explain the rationale for use of antianemia therapy.

- Identify the nursing implications during assessment, implementation, and evaluation of the patient receiving antianemic therapy.

- Discuss appropriate patient teaching for the patient receiving antianemia therapy.

- Name the common side effects of agents used to treat anemia.

XVII. The Patient with Anemia

A. Antianemia therapy: general information

1. Mechanism of action: depends on the type of anemia (see specific information)
2. Indications: to prevent or treat anemia
3. Contraindications: undiagnosed anemias, hemochromatosis, hemosiderosis, hemolytic anemia
4. Side effects: see specific information
5. Interactions: see specific information
6. Nursing implications
   a. Assessment: assess patient's nutritional status and dietary history to determine possible causes of anemia and need for patient teaching
   b. Evaluation: base on improved laboratory values
7. Patient teaching
   a. Emphasize the importance of a nutritionally balanced diet
   b. Emphasize the importance of compliance with the drug regimen

B. Iron products: specific information

1. Mechanism of action: supplement and replace iron stores
2. Indications: erythropoietic abnormalities due to deficiency of iron
3. Side effects
   a. Oral preparations: constipation, dark stools, diarrhea, GI distress
   b. Parenteral preparations: nausea, vomiting, headache, staining at I.M. site, anaphylaxis
4. Interactions: tetracyclines and antacids inhibit absorption and ascorbic acid increases absorption if given with oral iron preparations
5. Nursing implications
   a. Assessment: monitor hemoglobin, reticulocyte values, and plasma iron levels
   b. Implementation: administer oral preparations on an empty stomach unless GI distress occurs. Dilute liquid preparations and administer with a straw to prevent staining teeth. Give I.M. preparations via Z-track injection
   c. Evaluation: base on increased hemoglobin and plasma iron levels
6. Patient teaching
   a. Instruct patient to follow a diet high in iron
   b. Advise patient to avoid using antacids, coffee, tea, dairy products, eggs, or whole-grain breads 1 hour before and 2 hours after taking oral preparations
   c. Caution patient that stools may become dark green or black
7. Drug examples
   a. Ferrous gluconate (Fergon)
   b. Ferrous sulfate (Feosol)
   c. Iron dextran (Imferon)

C. Vitamins: specific information
  1. Indications
     a. Vitamin B_{12} deficiency (pernicious anemia): cyanocobalamin
     b. Folic acid deficiency: folic acid
  2. Side effects
     a. Cyanocobalamin: diarrhea, itching, rash
     b. Folic acid: allergic reaction, allergic bronchospasm
  3. Interactions
     a. Cyanocobalamin: decreased absorption occurs with alcohol, anticonvulsants, and aspirin
     b. Folic acid: high doses may increase metabolism of phenobarbital and phenytoin
  4. Drug examples
     a. Cyanocobalamin (Betalin 12)
     b. Folic acid (Folvite)

Points to Remember

Anemias may be caused by deficiencies of vitamins or minerals that impair the body's ability to manufacture red blood cells; treatment focuses on replacing the deficient substances.

Nursing assessment for the patient with anemia should include nutritional status and diet history to determine possible causes of the anemia and areas for patient teaching.

Tetracyclines and antacids inhibit absorption of iron products.

Ascorbic acid increases absorption of iron products if given with oral iron preparations.

Glossary

Erythropoiesis—the formation of red blood cells

Hemochromatosis—rare disorder of iron storage, characterized by excessive accumulation of iron in the body

Hemolytic anemia—anemia resulting from hemolysis, or the breakdown of red blood cells

Pernicious anemia—chronic anemia caused by the failure of the stomach to secrete enough intrinsic factor to ensure intestinal absorption of vitamin B_{12}

The Patient Requiring Antilipemics

Learning Objectives

After studying this section, the reader should be able to:

● List indications for the use of antilipemics.

● Name the common side effects of antilipemics.

● Identify the nursing implications during assessment, implementation, and evaluation of the patient receiving antilipemics.

● Discuss appropriate patient teaching for the patient receiving antilipemics.

XVIII. The Patient Requiring Antilipemics

A. **Antilipemics: general information**
1. Mechanism of action: lower cholesterol and/or triglycerides
2. Indications: elevated serum cholesterol triglycerides
3. Contraindications: hypersensitivity and pregnancy
4. Side effects: diarrhea, abdominal pain
5. Interactions: bile acid sequestrants (cholestyramine, colestipol) may bind vitamins and drugs
6. Nursing implications
   a. Assessment: monitor serum cholesterol and triglyceride levels
   b. Evaluation: base on a decrease in cholesterol and triglyceride levels
7. Patient teaching: inform patient that these medications should be used in conjunction with diet restrictions (fat, cholesterol, carbohydrates, alcohol), exercise, and smoking cessation

B. **Antilipemics: specific information**
1. Mechanism of action
   a. Bile acid sequestrants bind acids in the GI tract, increasing the clearance of cholesterol
   b. Clofibrate decreases the hepatic synthesis and accelerates the breakdown of low-density lipoproteins
2. Drug examples
   a. Cholestyramine (Questran)
   b. Colestipol (Colestid)
   c. Clofibrate (Atromid-S)

Points to Remember

Antilipemics are used to lower serum cholesterol and triglyceride levels.

Antilipemics are used with exercise and diet modification.

Antilipemics are contraindicated in pregnancy.

Antilipemics may bind vitamins and drugs.

Glossary

Antilipemic—drug that prevents or treats increased accumulation of fatty substances (lipids) in blood

Bile acid—steroid acid of bile, produced during cholesterol metabolism

Cholesterol—fat-soluble, crystalline steroid alcohol; found in egg yolks and animal fats

Triglyceride—chief lipid in blood; fatty acid-glycerol compound; makes up most animal and vegetable fats

The Patient Requiring Anticoagulation

Learning Objectives

After studying this section, the reader should be able to:

● Describe the difference between anticoagulants and thrombolytics.

● Describe the precautions necessary for the patient receiving anticoagulants.

● Identify the nursing implications during assessment, implementation, and evaluation of the patient receiving drugs for anticoagulation.

● Discuss appropriate patient teaching for the patient receiving drugs for anticoagulation.

● Identify the specific laboratory tests used to monitor the patient receiving heparin and warfarin.

XIX. The Patient Requiring Anticoagulation

A. **Anticoagulants/thrombolytics: general information**
  1. Mechanism of action
      a. Anticoagulants prevent clot extension and formation by inhibiting factors in the clotting cascade
      b. Thrombolytics activate plasminogen, converting it to plasmin, which degrades clots
  2. Indications: see specific information
  3. Contraindications: underlying coagulation disorders, ulcer disease, recent surgery, cancer, or active bleeding
  4. Side effects: bleeding
  5. Interactions: their use with other drugs affecting platelet function, including aspirin, nonsteroidal anti-inflammatory agents, dipyridamole, and dextran, may increase risk of bleeding
  6. Nursing implications
      a. Assessment: assess for bleeding and monitor clotting factors, platelet count, and hemoglobin
      b. Implementation: minimize venipunctures and injections. Apply pressure to all puncture sites
      c. Evaluation: base on prevention of clot formation and extension or breakdown of clots without side effects
  7. Patient teaching: advise patients to report signs and symptoms of bleeding immediately

B. **Anticoagulants: specific information**
  1. Indications: prevention and treatment of thromboembolic disorders, such as deep vein thrombosis, pulmonary embolism, and atrial fibrillation with embolization
  2. Side effects: heparin may cause thrombocytopenia
  3. Interactions: the effects of warfarin may be increased by androgens, chloramphenicol, chloral hydrate, metronidazole, thrombolytic agents, sulfonamides, quinidine, and valproic acid, and decreased by alcohol, barbiturates, estrogen-containing oral contraceptives, and foods high in vitamin K
  4. Nursing implications
      a. Heparin directly affects the partial thromboplastin time (PTT)
      b. Warfarin directly affects the prothrombin time (PT)
      c. Subcutaneous heparin is administered into the abdomen. Do not aspirate or rub site
      d. Patient is initially started on heparin because of its rapid action and then gradually converted to warfarin over a period of days
      e. The antidote for heparin is protamine sulfate
      f. The antidote for warfarin is phytonadione (AquaMEPHYTON; vitamin K)

5. Patient teaching
   a. Tell patient to use a soft toothbrush and an electric razor while on anticoagulant therapy
   b. Instruct patient to advise physicians and dentists of medication regimen before treatment
   c. Tell patient to include consistent amounts of vitamin K in diet
   d. Emphasize the importance of routine lab tests to monitor coagulation times
   e. Instruct patient to carry identification describing disease and drug regimen
6. Drug examples
   a. Heparin (Calciparine, Liquaemin, Panheprin)
   b. Warfarin (Coumadin)

C. **Thrombolytic agents: specific information**
   1. Indications: used to treat massive pulmonary emboli, deep vein thromboses; used in the lysis of coronary artery thrombi, arterial thrombi; and used to clear arterial catheters and AV cannuli
   2. Contraindications: streptokinase is contraindicated in recent streptococcal infections
   3. Side effects: urticaria, fever
   4. Nursing implications
      a. Thrombolytic agents should only be used in settings where hematologic function and clinical response can be monitored
      b. Monitor vital signs and peripheral pulses frequently
      c. Typed and crossmatched blood should be available in case of hemorrhage
      d. Aminocaproic acid (Amicar) is the antidote
   5. Drug examples
      a. Streptokinase (Kabikinase, Streptase)
      b. Urokinase (Abbokinase)

Points to Remember

Nursing responsibilities for the patient on anticoagulants include assessing for gross or occult bleeding, monitoring lab coagulation values, and implementing appropriate safety measures to prevent bleeding.

Anticoagulants are potent medications that may cause hemorrhage.

The antidote for heparin is protamine sulfate; the antidote for warfarin is vitamin K; the antidote for thrombolytic agents is aminocaproic acid.

The patient needing anticoagulation is usually started on heparin because of its rapid action, then gradually converted to oral anticoagulants, which take several days to reach an effective level.

Glossary

Anticoagulant—agent that prevents the formation or extension of clots. It does not speed the dissolution of preexisting clots, which occurs naturally in 7 days

Partial thromboplastin time (PTT)—diagnostic test for coagulation defects of the intrinsic system, except for Factors VII and XIII

Prothrombin time (PT)—diagnostic test for coagulation defects caused by deficiency of Factors V, VII, or X

Thrombolytic agent—agent that dissolves existing clots by activating plasminogen and converting it to plasmin, which dissolves clots

The Patient in Bronchospasm

Learning Objectives

After studying this section, the reader should be able to:

- Describe the mechanism of action of bronchodilators and anti-inflammatory agents.

- Explain the rationale for use of bronchodilators and anti-inflammatory agents.

- List the common side effects of bronchlodilators and anti-inflammatory agents.

- Identify the nursing implications during assessment, implementation, and evaluation of the patient receiving bronchodilators or anti-inflammatory agents.

- Discuss appropriate patient teaching for the patient receiving bronchodilators or anti-inflammatory agents.

XX. The Patient in Bronchospasm

A. Drugs for bronchospasm: general information

1. Mechanism of action
   a. Sympathomimetic agents (bronchodilators): produce bronchodilation by stimulating the production of cyclic adenosine monophosphate (cAMP)
   b. Phosphodiesterase inhibitors (bronchodilators): inhibit breakdown of cAMP
   c. Anti-inflammatory agents: prevent or counteract the biochemical mediators (kinins, serotonin, histamine) that cause tissue inflammation responsible for edema and narrowing of airways
2. Indications: to prevent or treat bronchospasm
3. Contraindications: uncontrolled cardiac dysrhythmias
4. Side effects: see specific information
5. Interactions: see specific information
6. Nursing implications
   a. Assessment: assess blood pressure, pulse, respiratory status, and lung sounds throughout administration
   b. Implementation: administer these drugs around the clock
   c. Evaluation: base on increased ease of breathing and clearing of lung fields on auscultation without side effects
7. Patient teaching
   a. Instruct patient on use of inhalation medications
   b. Explain that fluid intake of 2,000 to 3,000 ml/day is needed to decrease viscosity of secretions
   c. Advise patient to avoid over-the-counter drugs without consulting physician or pharmacist

B. Sympathomimetic agents (see Section II): specific information

1. Side effects
   a. Anxiety, nervousness, tremors, headache
   b. Palpitations, tachycardia, hypertension
2. Interactions
   a. These agents are antagonized by beta-blocking agents
   b. Additive effects occur with theophylline preparations
3. Drug examples
   a. Epinephrine (Adrenalin, Sus-Phrine)
   b. Isoproterenol (Isuprel)
   c. Metaproterenol (Metaprel, Alupent)
   d. Terbutaline (Brethaire, Brethine, Bricanyl)
   e. Albuterol (Ventolin, Proventil)

C. Phosphodiesterase inhibitors: specific information

1. Contraindications: shock, hypertension, seizures, active peptic ulcer, liver failure, GI bleeding, acute hyperthyroidism

2. Side effects
   a. Tachycardia, palpitations, dysrhythmias, hypotension, shock, possible hypertension
   b. Anorexia, nausea, cramps, indigestion, diarrhea, thirst
   c. Anxiety, dizziness, tremor, headache, insomnia, nervousness
3. Interactions
   a. These agents are antagonized by beta-blocking agents
   b. They are potentiated by sympathomimetics and cardiac glycosides
   c. Diuretics may potentiate diuretic effects
   d. Phenobarbital, phenytoin, rifampin, smoking, and eating charcoal-broiled foods may shorten the half-life
   e. These agents may reduce the effects of lithium
4. Nursing implications: monitor blood levels for toxicity; may cause dysrhythmias and seizures
5. Patient teaching
   a. Advise patient to minimize intake of xanthine-containing foods or beverages (cola, coffee, chocolate)
   b. Emphasize the importance of maintaining routine blood levels of these agents
6. Drug examples
   a. Aminophylline (Somophyllin)
   b. Theophylline (Constant-T, Elixophyllin, Slo-bid, Slo-Phyllin, Somophyllin-CRT, Theobid, Theo-Dur)

D. Anti-inflammatory agents: specific information
1. Indications
   a. Treatment of chronic bronchospasm (beclomethasone)
   b. Prevention of inflammation (cromolyn sodium)
2. Contraindications: acute bronchospasm
3. Side effects
   a. Hoarseness, oropharyngeal irritation, monilial infections (beclomethasone)
   b. Coughing, throat irritation, reactive bronchospasm (cromolyn sodium)
4. Patient teaching: tell the patient receiving bronchodilators and beclomethasone by inhalation to use bronchodilators several minutes before beclomethasone
5. Drug examples
   a. Beclomethasone (Vanceril, Beclovent, Beconase, Vancenase)
   b. Cromolyn sodium (Intal)

Points to Remember

Sympathomimetics and phosphodiesterase inhibitors produce bronchodilation by increasing cAMP; their major side effects include cardiac dysrhythmias, anxiety, tremors, and palpitations.

Many of these drugs are administered via various methods of inhalation; the patient must be taught the appropriate method of administration.

When taking respiratory drugs, the patient generally should increase fluids and avoid respiratory irritants.

Smoking, eating charcoal-broiled food, and taking certain medications may shorten the half-life of phosphodiesterase inhibitors such as aminophylline and theophylline.

Glossary

Auscultation—common assessment technique of listening for sounds within the body

Bronchospasm—narrowing of the bronchioles from an increase in smooth muscle tone; causes wheezing

Cyclic adenosine monophosphate (cAMP)—a nucleotide, produced by stimulation of the beta$_2$ receptors in the lungs, that causes bronchodilation when it is released

Inhalation medications—medications that affect the respiratory tract locally; may be administered by hand-held nebulizers, intermittent positive pressure breathing (IPPB), nasal sprays, or drops

The Patient with Increased Bronchial Secretions

Learning Objectives

After studying this section, the reader should be able to:

● Describe the mechanism of action of antitussives, expectorants, and mucolytics.

● Explain the rationale for use of antitussives, expectorants, and mucolytics.

● List the common side effects of antitussives, expectorants, and mucolytics.

● Identify the nursing implications during assessment, implementation, and evaluation of the patient receiving antitussives, expectorants, or mucolytics.

● Discuss appropriate patient teaching for the patient receiving antitussives, expectorants, or mucolytics.

XXI. The Patient with Increased Bronchial Secretions

A. **Antitussives, expectorants, mucolytics: general information**
  1. Mechanism of action
     a. Antitussives: suppress the cough reflex by acting on the cough center in the medulla
     b. Expectorants: reduce the viscosity of tenacious secretions by causing increased fluid in the respiratory tract
     c. Mucolytics: decrease mucus viscosity by breaking its structural bonds
  2. Indications
     a. Antitussives: nonproductive cough, or coughs that interfere with sleep or daily activities
     b. Expectorants and mucolytics: coughs with tenacious secretions
  3. Contraindications: see specific information
  4. Side effects: nausea
  5. Interactions: see specific information
  6. Nursing implications
     a. Assessment: assess lung sounds, frequency and type of cough, and character of bronchial secretions
     b. Implementation: fluid intake of 2,000 to 3,000 ml/day is needed to decrease viscosity of secretions
     c. Evaluation: base on decreased frequency of nonproductive coughs and decreased viscosity of secretions
  7. Patient teaching
     a. Advise patient with nonproductive coughs to minimize talking, stop smoking, maintain moisture in environmental air, and use gum or sugarless candy to minimize cough
     b. Tell patient to consult physician if cough persists longer than 1 week or is accompanied by fever or chest pain
     c. Advise patient not to take liquids within 30 minutes of antitussives because liquids may negate local soothing effects

B. **Antitussives: specific information**
  1. Side effects
     a. Narcotic antitussives: drowsiness, drying of respiratory secretions, constipation
     b. Non-narcotic antitussives: drowsiness, dizziness
  2. Interactions: potentiated by monoamine oxidase (MAO) inhibitors, alcohol, anticholinergics, sedatives, and tranquilizers
  3. Drug examples
     a. Narcotic antitussives: codeine, hydrocodone
     b. Non-narcotic antitussives: dextromethorphan (Hold, Romilar, Pertussin), diphenhydramine (Benadryl, Benalyn)

C. **Expectorants: specific information**
  1. Contraindications: do not use potassium iodide with patients allergic to iodine
  2. Drug examples
     a. Guaifenesin (Robitussin)
     2. Terpin hydrate
     3. Potassium iodide (SSKI)

D. **Mucolytics: specific information**
  1. Indications: acetylcysteine is also used as an antidote for acetaminophen overdose
  2. Drug example: acetylcysteine (Mucomyst)

Points to Remember

Antitussives are used only with a dry, nonproductive cough, or coughs that interfere with sleep or daily activities. They are not used with productive coughs.

The effect of expectorants is enhanced by increasing fluid intake to decrease the viscosity of pulmonary secretions.

Expectorants and mucolytics are used to treat coughs with tenacious secretions.

Mucolytics decrease mucus viscosity by breaking its structural bonds.

Glossary

Nonproductive cough—a dry, hacking cough that does not produce sputum

Potentiate—to increase the action of another drug; when this occurs, the combined effect of the two drugs is greater than the sum of the effect of each alone

Viscosity—state of being glutinous or sticky

The Patient with a Pituitary Disorder

Learning Objectives

After studying this section, the reader should be able to:

- Describe the mechanism of action of growth and antidiuretic hormones.

- Explain the rationale for the use of growth and antidiuretic hormones.

- List the major side effects of growth and antidiuretic hormones.

- Identify the nursing implications during assessment, implementation, and evaluation of the patient receiving growth or antidiuretic hormone.

- Discuss appropriate patient teaching for the patient receiving a growth or antidiuretic hormone.

XXII. The Patient with a Pituitary Disorder

A. **Growth hormone: general information**
1. Mechanism of action: causes increased rate of growth
2. Indications: pituitary dwarfism
3. Contraindications: closed epiphyses and intracranial tumors
4. Side effects: excessive doses may cause giantism in children
5. Interactions: corticosteroids, thyroid, estrogens, or androgens may precipitate epiphyseal closure
6. Nursing implications
    a. Assessment: monitor blood and urine glucose regularly
    b. Implementation: be aware that injection may cause pain and swelling
    c. Evaluation: base on increased height without side effects
7. Patient teaching: emphasize the importance of regular blood and urine glucose monitoring
8. Drug example: somatrem (Protropin)

B. **Antidiuretic hormone: general information**
1. Mechanism of action: enhances reabsorption of water in the kidneys. Vasopressin also causes vasoconstriction and decreased hepatic blood flow
2. Indications
    a. Diabetes insipidus (vasopressin, desmopressin)
    b. Control of bleeding in certain types of hemophilia (desmopressin)
    c. GI bleeding (vasopressin)
3. Contraindications: type IIB or platelet-type von Willebrand's disease (desmopressin)
4. Side effects: water intoxication, abdominal cramps, nausea, nasal congestion, flushing, hypertension, chest pain
5. Interactions
    a. Decreased response with lithium, epinephrine, heparin, alcohol, and demeclocycline
    b. Increased response with chlorpropamide, clofibrate, urea, and fludrocortisone
6. Nursing implications
    a. Assessment: monitor intake and output and urine osmolality frequently
    b. Evaluation: base on decreased urine volume and increased urine osmolality
7. Patient teaching
    a. Instruct patient on correct method of intranasal use
    b. Advise patient to consult physician if he has rhinitis or nasal congestion because they may decrease effect of intranasal therapy
    c. Warn against alcohol use with these medications
8. Drug examples
    a. Vasopressin (Pitressin, Pitressin Tannate)
    b. Desmopressin (DDAVP, Stimate)

Points to Remember

The pituitary gland secretes growth hormone.

Antidiuretic hormone is secreted by the hypothalamus and stored in the pituitary gland.

Children taking growth hormone should have their bone age determined annually.

Antidiuretic hormone, also called vasopressin, can be taken intranasally.

Glossary

Bone age—determination of the stage of development of the ossification centers of long bones where cartilage is replaced with true bone as the child develops

Epiphysis—the end of a long bone that is separated from the shaft by a cartilaginous disk (epiphyseal plate) until growth stops

Pituitary dwarfism—form of dwarfism caused by deficient growth hormone, which is produced by the anterior pituitary gland

Von Willebrand's disease—inherited coagulation disorder, occurring equally in males and females, characterized by prolonged bleeding time, spontaneous nosebleeds, and gingival bleeding; caused by deficiency of Factor VIII

The Patient Requiring Adrenocortical Drugs

Learning Objectives

After studying this section, the reader should be able to:

- Describe the mechanism of action of adrenocortical drugs.

- Explain the indications for adrenocortical drugs.

- List the common side effects of adrenocortical drugs.

- Identify the nursing implications during assessment, implementation, and evaluation of the patient receiving adrenocortical drugs

- Discuss appropriate patient teaching for the patient receiving adrenocortical drugs.

XXIII. The Patient Requiring Adrenocortical Drugs

A. **Adrenal cortical drugs: general information**
 1. Mechanism of action
     a. Mineralocorticoids enhance the reabsorption of sodium and chloride and the excretion of potassium and hydrogen from the kidney tubules
     b. Glucocorticoids produce varied metabolic effects, suppress inflammation, and alter the normal immune response
 2. Indications: see specific information
 3. Contraindications and precautions
     a. Use mineralocorticoids with caution in patients with cardiovascular disease or hypertension
     b. Use glucocorticoids with extreme caution in patients with serious infections
 4. Side effects: sodium and water retention, hypokalemia
 5. Interactions: additive hypokalemia with potassium-depleting diuretics and other drugs causing hypokalemia
 6. Nursing implications: see specific information
 7. Patient teaching: see specific information

B. **Mineralocorticoids: specific information**
 1. Indications: replacement therapy for patient with primary and secondary adrenal insufficiency
 2. Patient teaching: instruct patient to eat a high-potassium diet
 3. Drug examples
     a. Desoxycorticosterone (DOCA, Percorten)
     b. Fludrocortisone (Florinef)

C. **Glucocorticoids: specific information**
 1. Indications
     a. Replacement therapy for adrenal cortical insufficiency
     b. Inflammation (joint, GI, respiratory, skin)
     c. Neoplastic diseases
     d. Septic shock
     e. Autoimmune diseases
     f. Cerebral edema
 2. Side effects
     a. Muscle wasting, osteoporosis, growth retardation in children, fragile skin; may mask signs of infection
     b. Peptic ulcer
     c. Increased blood sugar, hypertension
     d. Mood swings, cataracts, glaucoma, convulsions
     e. Hirsutism, altered fat distribution
 3. Interactions
     a. These agents may increase requirement for insulin or oral hypoglycemics

      b. Phenytoin, phenobarbital, and rifampin may decrease effectiveness

      c. Oral contraceptives may block metabolism

4. Nursing implications

      a. Assessment: assess patient for improvement or worsening of disease symptomatology and for side effects

      b. Implementation: administer daily doses in the morning to correspond with the body's normal secretion of cortisol. Additional doses may be needed during stress

      c. Evaluation: base on improvement in presenting symptoms with minimal side effects

5. Patient teaching

      a. Emphasize the importance of compliance. Stopping abruptly may cause life-threatening adrenal insufficiency

      b. Tell patient to avoid vaccinations without consulting physician

      c. Advise patient to carry identification describing disease and medication regimen

6. Drug examples

      a. Cortisone (Cortone)

      b. Hydrocortisone (Hydrocortone, Solu-Cortef)

      c. Methylprednisolone (Medrol, Depo-Medrol, Solu-Medrol)

      d. Prednisone (Deltasone, Medicorten)

      e. Triamcinolone (Aristocort)

      f. Dexamethasone (Decadron, Hexadrol)

Points to Remember

The adrenal cortex normally secretes mineralocorticoids and glucocorticoids.

The patient taking mineralocorticoids or glucocorticoids should follow a high-potassium diet because these drugs enhance the excretion of potassium.

Glucocorticoids should be used with extreme caution in the patient with a serious infection.

A higher incidence of side effects occurs when hormones, such as the glucocorticoids, are given in doses above normal body levels for nonendocrine disorders than when they are given for replacement therapy.

Glucocorticoids must never be stopped abruptly because adrenal insufficiency may result; dosage must be weaned slowly.

Glossary

Adrenocortical—referring to adrenal cortex, the largest portion of the adrenal gland, which produces androgens, glucocorticoids, mineralocorticoids, and other hormones

Glucocorticoid—hormone secreted by the adrenal cortex that increases formation of carbohydrates from noncarbohydrate molecules and exerts an anti-inflammatory effect, among its many functions

Hirsutism—excessive body hair

Mineralocorticoid—hormone secreted by the adrenal cortex that maintains normal blood volume and promotes sodium retention and urinary excretion of potassium

The Patient Requiring Male or Female Hormones

Learning Objectives

After studying this section, the reader should be able to:

- Describe the mechanism of action for male and female hormones.

- Explain the indications for use of male and female hormones.

- List the common side effects of male and female hormones.

- Identify the nursing implications during assessment, implementation, and evaluation of the patient receiving male or female hormones.

- Discuss appropriate patient teaching for the patient receiving male or female hormones.

XXIV. The Patient Requiring Male or Female Hormones

A. Male hormones: general information
1. Mechanism of action: replace deficient hormones or treat hormone-sensitive disorders
2. Indications: see specific information
3. Contraindications: pregnancy, lactation, cancer of the prostate or male breast, prostatic hypertrophy, liver or cardiac disease
4. Side effects
    a. Nausea, vomiting, diarrhea, weight gain, mood swings
    b. Sodium and water retention, edema, changes in libido
    c. In boys: precocious puberty, priapism, premature epiphyseal closure
    d. In men: breast tenderness, impotence, sterility
    e. In females: hirsutism, reduced breast size, hoarseness
5. Interactions
    a. Use of male hormones with glucocorticoids increases edema
    b. Androgens may cause increased effects of oral anticoagulants, insulins, and oral hypoglycemics
6. Nursing implications
    a. Assessment: assess patient for weight gain and edema
    b. Evaluation: base on resolution of signs of androgen deficiency or symptoms of hormone-sensitive disorders
7. Patient teaching
    a. Emphasize the importance of compliance
    b. Tell patient to use nonhormonal contraception during therapy

B. Androgens: specific information
1. Indications
    a. Androgen deficiency, postpartum breast engorgement, palliative treatment of androgen-sensitive breast cancer (testosterone)
    b. Endometriosis, palliative treatment of fibrocystic breast disease, prophylaxis of hereditary angioedema (danazol)
2. Patient teaching: Tell female patient on danazol to expect amenorrhea
3. Drug examples
    a. Testosterone (Oreton, Depo-Test, Delatestryl)
    b. Danazol (Danocrine)

C. Anabolic steroids: specific information
1. Indications
    a. Catabolic disorders (infections, surgery, trauma)
    b. Anemia
    c. Arthritis, osteoporosis
    d. Palliative treatment of breast cancer
2. Drug examples
    a. Nandrolone (Durabolin, Deca-Durabolin)
    b. Oxandrolone (Anavar)

D. Female hormones: general information
  1. Mechanism of action
     a. Estrogens and progestogens restore hormonal balance in deficiency and treat hormone-sensitive tumors
     b. Lactation suppressants decrease serum prolactin levels
     c. Fertility medications increase levels of pituitary gonadotropins, which stimulate ovarian function
     d. Oxytoxics enhance uterine motility
     e. Labor suppressants relax uterine muscles and decrease uterine contractions
  2. Indications: see specific information
  3. Contraindications
     a. Estrogens and progestogens are contraindicated in thrombophlebitis or embolism, history of cerebral vascular accident, and breast neoplasms. They should be used cautiously with asthma, epilepsy, migraine, cardiac and renal disease
     b. Oxytoxics are contraindicated in obstetric emergencies, maternal hypertension, and toxemia
  4. Side effects: see specific information
  5. Interactions: see specific information
  6. Nursing implications: see specific information
  7. Patient teaching: see specific information

E. Estrogens and progestogens: specific information
  1. Indications
     a. Hormonal deficiencies
     b. Contraception
     c. Dysmenorrhea and dysfunctional uterine bleeding
     d. Hot flashes and atropic vaginitis during menopause (estrogens)
     e. Postcoital contraception (diethylstilbestrol)
     f. Restoration of positive calcium balance in postmenopausal osteoporosis (estrogen)
     g. Cancer: breast (estrogen), prostatic (diethylstilbestrol)
     h. Endometriosis (estrogen)
  2. Side effects
     a. Nausea, vomiting, diarrhea, weight gain, edema, rash
     b. Headache, insomnia, hypertension
  3. Interactions
     a. Effects of estrogens are decreased with barbiturates, penicillins, sulfonamides, and tetracyclines
     b. Estrogens decrease the effects or oral anticoagulants, anticonvulsants, and antidiabetic drugs
  4. Nursing implications
     a. Assessment: assess patient for edema and monitor blood pressure and weight

   b. Evaluation: base on contraception or resolution of symptoms without side effects
5. Patient teaching
   a. Instruct patient on correct technique for administration (oral, intravaginal, transdermal)
   b. Emphasize the importance of compliance with therapy
   c. Warn against cigarette smoking; it increases risk of side effects, especially in women over age 35
   d. Inform patient that routine breast, pelvic, and blood pressure examinations and Pap smears are necessary
6. Drug examples
   a. Diethylstilbestrol (DES, Stilbestrol)
   b. Conjugated estrogens (Premarin)
   c. Estradiol (Aquadiol, Depo-Estradiol, Delestrogen)
   d. Medoxyprogesterone acetate (Provera)
   e. Progesterone (Gesterol, Lipo-Luten)
   f. Norethindrone/mestranol (Norinyl, Ortho-Novum)

F. Lactation suppressants: specific information
1. Indications: reduce breast engorgement in the postpartum period and inhibit the secretion of prolactin in pituitary tumors
2. Drug examples
   a. Estradiol (Deladumone OB)
   b. Bromocriptine (Parlodel)

G. Fertility Medications: specific information
1. Indications: infertility from anovulation
2. Side effects: multiple births
3. Drug examples
   a. Human chorionic gonadotropins (HCG, Follutein)
   b. Menotropins (Pergonal)
   c. Clomiphene (Clomid)

H. Oxytocics: specific information
1. Indications
   a. Facilitate labor
   b. Manage postpartum hemorrhage
   c. Test uteroplacental respiratory reserve
   d. Induce therapeutic abortion through the second trimester of pregnancy
2. Side effects
   a. Nausea, vomiting, bradycardia, hypertension, anaphylaxis
   b. Fetal: bradycardia, hypoxia, intracranial hemorrhage; maternal: tetanic contractions, dysrhythmias (oxytocin)
3. Nursing implications: monitor blood pressure, pulse, output, contractions, vaginal bleeding, and fetal heart rate

   4. Drug examples
       a. Oxytocin (Pitocin, Syntocinon)
       b. Ergonovine maleate (Ergotrate)
       c. Methylergonovine maleate (Methergine)

I. Labor suppressants: specific information
   1. Indications: premature labor occurring between the 29th and 36th weeks of gestation
   2. Contraindications: ruptured membranes, abruptio placentae, hypertension, preeclampsia, fetal distress, pregnancy of less than 20 weeks
   3. Side effects: maternal widening pulse pressure and tachycardia
   4. Nursing implications: place the patient on her left side to allow venous return to the heart and decrease hypotension. Monitor patient and fetus closely. Usually begin with I.V. administration and change to oral administration when stable
   5. Drug example: ritodrine (Yutopar)

Points to Remember

Some hormonal agents replace hormone deficits whereas others, such as the fertility drugs, stimulate the endocrine gland to produce more of the hormone.

Side effects reflect overactivity or underactivity of the respective gland.

Fertility medications increase levels of pituitary gonadotropins, which stimulate ovarian function.

Multiple births are a possible side effect of fertility medication.

Glossary

Anovulation—the lack of production or discharge of an ovum

Endometriosis—abnormal conditon characterized by ectopic growth and function of endometrium

Priapism—abnormal, painful, prolonged or constant penile erection, usually without sexual desire; associated with disease

Widening pulse pressure—an increase in the difference between the systolic and diastolic blood pressures

The Patient with a Thyroid Disorder

Learning Objectives

After studying this section, the reader should be able to:

- Describe the mechanism of action of thyroid hormone and antithyroid medication.

- Explain the indications for thyroid hormone and antithyroid medication.

- List the common side effects of thyroid hormone and antithyroid medication.

- Identify the nursing implications during assessment, implementation, and evaluation of the patient receiving thyroid hormone or antithyroid medication.

- Discuss appropriate patient teaching for the patient receiving thyroid hormone or antithyroid medication.

XXV. The Patient with a Thyroid Disorder

A. Thyroid hormone: general information

1. Mechanism of action: controls the metabolic rate of tissues and accelerates heat production and oxygen consumption. Synthetic compounds have same physiologic effects as natural hormones
2. Indications: see specific information
3. Contraindications and precautions
    a. Thyroid hormone is contraindicated with thyrotoxicosis
    b. It is used with caution in cardiac disease and hypertension
4. Side effects: tachycardia, nervousness, sweating, heat intolerance, insomnia, weight loss, dysrhythmias
5. Interactions
    a. Aspirin and phenytoin potentiate effects
    b. Thyroid hormone decreases effects of stimulants and oral anticoagulants
6. Nursing implications
    a. Assessment: monitor thyroid function studies and pulse
    b. Implementation: administer in the morning to prevent insomnia
    c. Evaluation: base on normal thyroid levels, weight loss, increased appetite, pulse rate, energy, and sense of well-being
7. Patient teaching
    a. Tell patient not to change brands because different brands have different potencies
    b. Emphasize the importance of compliance with therapy

B. Thyroid hormone: specific information

1. Indications
    a. Replacement of thyroid hormone deficiency
    b. Simple goiter
2. Drug examples
    a. Thyroid USP (Thyrocrine)
    b. Liotrix (Euthroid, Thyrolar)
    c. Levothyroxine (Synthroid)
    d. Liothyronine (Cytomel)

C. Antithyroid medications: general information

1. Mechanism of action: inhibit the synthesis of thyroid hormones
2. Indications
    a. Hyperthyroidism (Graves' disease)
    b. To decrease symptoms and thyroid friability before surgery
3. Contraindications: pregnancy and lactation
4. Side effects: see specific information
5. Interactions
    a. Antithyroid medications may enhance anticoagulants (propylthiouracil, methimazole)

       b. Their use with lithium may potentiate hypothyroidism
6. Nursing implications
       a. Assessment: monitor thyroid levels and assess patient for signs of overdosage (hypothyroidism) or underdosage (thyrotoxicosis)
       b. Implementation: because food may affect absorption administer at a consistent time in relation to meals
       c. Evaluation: base on normal thyroid levels, weight loss, and lowered pulse rate
7. Patient teaching
       a. Tell patient to monitor weight weekly
       b. Instruct patient to consult physician regarding dietary sources of iodine
       c. Instruct patient to avoid aspirin and medications containing iodine
       d. Emphasize the importance of compliance and routine follow-up

D. Antithyroid medications: specific information
1. Side effects
       a. Rash, nausea, vomiting, agranulocytosis (propylthiouracil, methimazole)
       b. Hypothyroidism, diarrhea, hypersensitivity (iodine)
       c. Iodism: vomiting, abdominal pain, metallic taste, rash, sore salivary glands (iodine)
2. Drug examples
       a. Propylthiouracil (PTU)
       b. Methimazole (Tapazole)
       c. Strong iodine solution (Lugol's solution)

Points to Remember

Drugs used in hormonal disorders either replace hormone deficits or suppress excess hormone production.

Synthetic thyroid hormones have the same physiologic effect as the natural hormone.

Thyroid hormone should be administered in the morning to prevent insomnia.

The patient taking an antithyroid medication should avoid aspirin and medications containing iodine.

Glossary

Goiter—enlarged thyroid gland, usually manifested as a swelling in the neck

Hyperthyroidism—disorder caused by oversecretion of the thyroid gland, characterized by increased metabolism and goiter

Hypothyroidism—disorder caused by undersecretion of the thyroid gland, characterized by decreased metabolism, fatigue, and cold sensitivity

Thyrotoxicosis—a toxic condition resulting from hyperactivity of the thyroid gland that causes rapid heart rate, tremors, elevated basal metabolism, enlarged thyroid gland, exophthalmos, nervousness, and weight loss

The Patient with a Parathyroid Disorder

Learning Objectives

After studying this section, the reader should be able to:

- Describe the mechanism of action of parathyroid and antihypercalcemic drugs.

- Explain the indications for parathyroid and antihypercalcemic drugs.

- List the common side effects of parathyroid and antihypercalcemic drugs.

- Identify the nursing implications during assessment, implementation, and evaluation of the patient receiving parathyroid or antihypercalcemic drugs.

- Discuss appropriate patient teaching for the patient receiving parathyroid or antihypercalcemic drugs.

XXVI. The Patient with a Parathyroid Disorder

A. Drugs for parathyroid disorders: general information
   1. Mechanism of action
       a. Parathyroid drugs increase serum calcium and decrease serum phosphate levels
       b. Antihypercalcemic drugs lower serum calcium levels
   2. Indications: see specific information
   3. Contraindications: parathyroid drugs are contraindicated in hypercalcemia and used cautiously in renal failure
   4. Side effects: see specific information
   5. Interactions
       a. Use of calcium salts with digitalis increases the risk of digitalis toxicity
       b. Use of parathyroid drugs with magnesium-containing antacids may cause hypermagnesemia
       c. Oral calcium salts decrease absorption of tetracyclines
       d. Vitamin D enhances absorption of calcium
   6. Nursing implications
       a. Assessment: monitor electrolyte levels and assess patient for signs of hypocalcemia and hypercalcemia
       b. Evaluation: base on normal serum calcium level
   7. Patient teaching: tell the patient on oral calcium preparations to avoid excessive amounts of spinach, whole grains, and rhubarb and to maintain an adequate intake of calcium and vitamin D

B. Drugs for parathyroid disorders: specific information
   1. Indications
       a. Parathyroid drugs: hypocalcemia, hypoparathyroidism
       b. Antihypercalcemic drugs: hypercalcemia, Paget's disease
   2. Side effects
       a. Parathyroid drugs: hypercalcemia (nausea, vomiting, anorexia, polyuria, polydipsia, constipation, dysrhythmias, weakness, calculi, lethargy)
       b. Antihypercalcemic drugs: hypocalcemia (nausea, vomiting, facial flushing, tetany, positive Trousseau's and Chvostek's signs)
   3. Drug examples
       a. Parathyroid drugs: calcitriol (Rocaltrol), calcium chloride, calcium gluconate, calcium lactate
       b. Antihypercalcemic drugs: calcitonin (Calcimar)

Points to Remember

The parathyroid gland secretes parathyroid hormone, which helps maintain serum calcium and phosphate levels.

The patient taking drugs for a parathyroid disorder should be assessed for signs of hypocalcemia and hypercalcemia.

The patient taking oral calcium preparations should avoid excessive amounts of spinach, whole grains, and rhubarb because these foods are high in calcium.

Agents used in parathyroid disorders are not hormones or hormone supplements, but are the minerals regulated by the parathyroid gland.

Glossary

Chvostek's sign—spasms of the facial muscles that result from tapping one side of the face over the facial nerve; indicates hypocalcemic tetany

Paget's disease—a chronic, progressive bone disorder

Parathyroid gland—four small glands that secrete parathyroid hormone, which regulates calcium and phosphorus metabolism

Trousseau's sign—muscle spasm of the arm that results from applying pressure to the upper arm with, for example, a blood pressure cuff; usually indicates hypocalcemic tetany

The Patient with Diabetes Mellitus

Learning Objectives

After studying this section, the reader should be able to:

- Describe the mechanism of action of insulin and oral hypoglycemic agents.

- Explain the rationale for use of insulin and oral hypoglycemic agents for the patient with diabetes mellitus.

- List the onset, peak, and duration of rapid-acting, intermediate-acting, and long-acting insulins.

- Identify the nursing implications during assessment, implementation, and evaluation of the patient receiving insulin or oral hypoglycemic agents.

- Discuss appropriate patient teaching for the patient receiving insulin or oral hypoglycemic agents.

XXVII. The Patient with Diabetes Mellitus

A. **Drugs for diabetes mellitus: general information**
 1. Mechanism of action
    a. Insulin increases the transport of glucose into cells and promotes the conversion of glucose to glycogen in order to lower blood sugar
    b. Oral hypoglycemic agents stimulate the pancreas to produce more insulin and increase peripheral receptors' sensitivity to insulin
 2. Indications: diabetes mellitus
 3. Contraindications and precautions
    a. Patients may be allergic to particular types of insulin
    b. Oral hypoglycemic agents in Type I or insulin-dependent diabetes mellitus (IDDM) should not be used
 4. Side effects: hypoglycemia
 5. Interactions
    a. Beta-adrenergic blocking agents may mask the symptoms of hypoglycemia
    b. Alcohol, glucocorticoids, thiazide diuretics, thyroid preparations, rifampin, and estrogens may increase insulin requirements and decrease the effectiveness of oral hypoglycemic agents
    c. Anabolic steroids, anticoagulants, salicylates, sulfonamides, monoamine oxidase (MAO) inhibitors, and chloramphenicol may require a reduction of insulin dosage and may increase the hypoglycemic effects of oral hypoglycemic agents
 6. Nursing implications
    a. Assessment: monitor blood or urine glucose and ketones. Assess patient for signs of hypoglycemia or hyperglycemia
    b. Implementation: be aware that patients exposed to stress, fever, trauma, infection, or surgery may require increased insulin doses or a conversion to insulin from oral hypoglycemic agents. Severe hypoglycemia may be treated with I.V. glucose or glucagon
    c. Evaluation: base on normal serum glucose levels without signs and symptoms of hypoglycemia or hyperglycemia
 7. Patient teaching
    a. Explain to patient that these medications control but do not cure diabetes; therapy is long-term
    b. Emphasize the importance of dietary compliance with diabetic diet and exchange system
    c. Instruct the patient on correct technique for monitoring blood or urine glucose
    d. Discuss the importance of regular exercise, daily examination of feet, and the avoidance of alcohol with these drugs
    e. Tell patient to contact physician if unable to eat or if blood or urine sugar levels are not controlled
    f. Instruct patient on the symptoms of hypoglycemia and hyperglycemia and what to do if they occur

    g. Tell patient to carry sugar and identification describing disease and drug therapy

B. Insulins: specific information
1. Indications
   a. Insulin-dependent diabetes mellitus (IDDM)
   b. Non-insulin-dependent diabetes mellitus (NIDDM) unresponsive to diet and oral hypoglycemic agents
2. Side effects
   a. Rebound hyperglycemia (Somogyi effect)
   b. Lipodystrophy
3. Nursing implications
   a. Use only insulin syringes. Check dose with another nurse before administering
   b. Draw regular insulin into syringe first when mixing insulins to avoid contamination of regular insulin vial
   c. Do not shake insulin vials; rotate between hands
   d. Remember that only regular insulin can be administered I.V.
   e. Schedule snacks for the time the patient is most likely to become hypoglycemic; may be at risk at more than one time if using a combination of insulins
   f. Keep insulin in a cool place
4. Patient teaching: instruct patient on correct technique for administration, rotation of sites, and disposal of used syringes
5. Drug examples
   a. Rapid-acting insulins: regular (Regular Ilentin I, Actrapid, Humulin R, Novolin R, Velosulin), prompt insulin zinc suspension (Semilente Ilentin I, Semitard)
   b. Intermediate-acting insulins: isophane insulin suspension (NPH Ilentin I(Humulin N, Insulatard NPH), insulin zinc suspension (Lente Ilentin I, Lentard, Monotard)
   c. Long-acting insulins: extended insulin zinc suspension (Ultralente Ilentin I, Ultratard), protamine zinc suspension (PZI, Protamine Zinc Ilentin I)
   d. Mixed insulins: 30% regular, 70% NPH (Mixtard)

C. Oral hypoglycemic agents: specific information
1. Indications: NIDDM when diet and exercise alone do not control blood sugar
2. Contraindications and precautions
   a. Use requires caution during pregnancy and lactation
   b. Patients allergic to sulfa drugs may also be allergic to oral hypoglycemic agents

3. Side effects
   a. Nausea, vomiting, heartburn
   b. Dizziness, drowsiness, headache, photosensitivity
4. Interactions: concurrent use of alcohol and oral hypoglycemic agents may cause a disulfiram-like reaction (abdominal cramps, nausea, vomiting, flushing, headache, hypoglycemia)
5. Patient teaching: tell patient to use sunscreen and protective clothing to prevent photosensitivity reactions
6. Drug examples
   a. Acetohexamide (Dymelor)
   b. Chlorpropamide (Diabinese, Glucamide)
   c. Glipizide (Glucotrol)
   d. Glyburide (Diabeta, Micronase)
   e. Tolazamide (Ronase, Tolinase)
   f. Tolbutamide (Orinase)

INSULIN COMPARISON CHART

TYPE	GENERIC NAME	TRADE NAME	ONSET OF ACTION (HRS)	PEAK CONCEN-TRATION LEVELS	DURATION OF ACTION
Rapid-acting	Insulin injection* (Regular)	Regular Iletin I, Actrapid, Humulin R, Novolin R, Velosulin	½ to 1	2 to 3	5 to 7
	Prompt insulin zinc suspension (Semilente)	Semilente Iletin I, Semitard	½ to 2	4 to 7	12 to 16
Intermediate-acting	Isophane insulin suspension (NPH)	NPH Iletin I, Humulin N, Insulatard NPH	1 to 2	8 to 12	24
	Insulin zinc suspension (Lente)	Lente Iletin I, Lentard, Monotard	1 to 2	8 to 12	24
Long-acting	Extended insulin zinc, suspension (Ultralente)	Ultralente Iletin I, Ultratard	4 to 8	16 to 18	36
	Protamine zinc insulin, suspension (PZI)	Protamine Zinc Iletin I	4 to 8	14 to 20	36

* Only *insulin injection, regular* may be administered by the I.V. route.

Note: Onset of action, peak concentration levels, duration of action times are based on subcutaneous (S.C.) administration route.

Points to Remember

Insulin increases the transport of glucose into cells and promotes the conversion of glucose to glycogen in order to lower blood sugar.

Insulin is used in the treatment of insulin-dependent diabetes mellitus (IDDM) and non-insulin-dependent diabetes mellitus (NIDDM) that is unresponsive to diet and oral hypoglycemic agents.

Oral hypoglycemic agents stimulate the pancreas to produce more insulin. They are used in the treatment of non-insulin-dependent diabetes mellitus (NIDDM) when diet and exercise alone do not control blood glucose.

Patient teaching for the patient with diabetes mellitus should include the symptoms of hypoglycemia and hyperglycemia and information on diet, exercise, foot care, and sick-day rules.

Glossary

Hyperglycemia—blood glucose above the normal level that produces drowsiness, flushed dry skin, fruitlike breath odor, frequent urination, fatigue, and unusual thirst

Hypoglycemia—blood glucose below the normal level that produces anxiety, chills, cold sweats, confusion, cool pale skin, difficulty concentrating, drowsiness, excessive hunger, headache, irritability, nervousness, nausea, rapid pulse, unusual fatigue or weakness

Lipodystrophy—thickening of tissues and accumulation of fat at the injection site caused by injecting insulin in the same site too frequently, injecting insulin too superficially, or injecting cold insulin

Somogyi effect—rebound hyperglycemia caused by excessive insulin dosage

The Patient with a Systemic Bacterial Infection

Learning Objectives

After studying this section, the reader should be able to:

● Summarize the general characteristics of the following drug families: penicillins, cephalosporins, aminoglycosides, and tetracyclines.

● List common side effects of these antibacterial agents.

● Differentiate among the general characteristics of the antibacterial agents.

● Identify the nursing implications during assessment, implementation, and evaluation of the patient receiving antibacterial agents.

● Discuss appropriate patient teaching for the patient receiving antibacterial agents.

XXVIII. The Patient with a Systemic Bacterial Infection

A. Antibacterials: general information

1. Mechanism of action: kill or inhibit the growth of susceptible bacteria. Categorized according to chemical similarities or antimicrobial spectrum
2. Indications: to treat or prevent bacterial infections
3. Contraindications: hypersensitivity
4. Side effects: use of broad-spectrum agents may lead to resistant bacteria and fungal superinfections
5. Interactions: see specific information
6. Nursing implications
   a. Assessment: assess patient for signs of infection. Specimens for culture and sensitivity should be obtained before initiating therapy; first dose may be given before receiving results
   b. Implementation: administer around the clock to maintain therapeutic blood levels
   c. Evaluation: base on resolution of signs and symptoms of infection
7. Patient teaching
   a. Emphasize the importance of compliance with therapy and completion of the full course of medication to prevent resistant bacterial strains
   b. Caution patient that sharing antibacterials may be dangerous
   c. Instruct patient to report signs of superinfection (black, furry overgrowth on tongue; loose or foul-smelling stools; vaginal itching or discharge) to physician

B. Penicillins: specific information

1. Indications: generally active against gram-positive cocci and bacilli and some gram-negative cocci
   a. Original penicillins: also effective against most anaerobes; drugs of choice for treating gonorrhea
   b. Penicillinase-resistant penicillins: primarily used to treat infections caused by staphylococci that synthesize the enzyme penicillinase
   c. Broad-spectrum penicillins: active against many organisms; used especially for enterococcal infections
   d. Extended-spectrum penicillins: increased activity against gram-negative bacteria
2. Contraindications
   a. Patient allergic to any penicillin or cephalosporin may be cross-sensitive to other drugs in this group
   b. Patients allergic to "caine-type" local anesthetics may be allergic to procaine penicillin G
3. Side effects
   a. Rash, anaphylaxis
   b. Nausea, vomiting, diarrhea, epigastric distress
   c. Pain at injection site, phlebitis at I.V. site

4. Interactions
    a. Extended-spectrum penicillins may inhibit platelet aggregation and may potentiate bleeding with other similar drugs
    b. Penicillins may decrease effectiveness of oral contraceptives
    c. Probenecid decreases renal excretion and increases blood levels of penicillins
    d. Penicillins may reduce the effectiveness of concurrently administered aminoglycosides
5. Nursing implications
    a. Obtain a careful patient history. Patients with a negative history of sensitivity may still have an allergic resonse
    b. Observe for signs of anaphylaxis. Discontinue the drug and notify physician if they occur
6. Patient teaching
    a. Tell patient to avoid taking oral penicillins with acidic juices or carbonated beverages because this may decrease absorption
    b. Tell patient allergic to penicillins to carry an identification card with this information
7. Drug examples
    a. Original penicillins: penicillin G (Pentids), penicillin V (Pen Vee K, V-Cillin)
    b. Penicillinase-resistant penicillins: cloxacillin (Tegopen), dicloxacillin (Dynapen), methicillin (Staphcillin), nafcillin (Unipen), oxacillin (Prostaphlin)
    c. Broad-spectrum penicillins: ampicillin, amoxicillin (Amoxil)
    d. Extended-release penicillins: carbenicillin (Geopen), azlocillin (Azlin), mezlocillin (Mezlin), piperacillin (Pipracil), ticarcillin (Ticar)

C. **Cephalosporins: specific information**
    1. Indications: active against gram-positive and gram-negative bacteria. First-generation cephalosporins are active against most gram-positive cocci and certain gram-negative bacilli. Each additional generation of cephalosporins has increased activity against gram-negative organism and decrease effectiveness against gram-positive organisms
    2. Contraindications and precautions: may have cross-sensitivity in patients allergic to penicillins
    3. Side effects
        a. Rash, anaphylaxis
        b. Nausea, vomiting, diarrhea
        c. Pain at I.M. site, phlebitis at I.V. site
    4. Interactions
        a. Probenecid decreases excretion and increases blood levels
        b. Cephalosporins may potentiate nephrotoxicity of other nephrotoxic drugs
        c. Concurrent use of alcohol with cefamandole, cefotetan, cefoperazone, or moxalactam may cause a disulfiram-like reaction (flushing, headache, tachycardia)

5. Nursing implications
   a. Obtain a careful patient history. Patients with a negative history of sensitivity may still have an allergic respone
   b. Observe for signs of anaphylaxis. Discontinue the drug and notify physician if they occur
   c. Use glucose oxidase reagent (Clinistix or Tes-Tape) to treat urine glucose; may cause false positive urine glucose results when tested with copper sulfate method (Clinitest)
6. Drug examples
   a. First generation: cefadroxil (Duricef), cefazolin (Ancef), cephalexin (Keflex), cephalothin (Keflin), cephapirin (Cefadyl), cephradine (Anspor, Velosef)
   b. Second generation: cefaclor (Ceclor), cefamandole (Mandol), cefonicid (Monocid), ceforanide (Precef), cefotetan (Cefotan), cefoxitin (Mefoxin), cefuroxime (Zinacef)
   c. Third generation: cefoperazone (Cefobid), cefotaxime (Claforan), ceftazidime (Fortaz, Tazicef, Tazidime), ceftizoxime (Cefizox), ceftriaxone (Rocephin), moxalactam (Moxam)

D. Aminoglycosides: specific information

1. Indications: primarily used to treat infections caused by aerobic gram-negative bacilli
2. Contraindications and precautions: use cautiously in renal failure and neuromuscular diseases
3. Side effects
   a. Ototoxicity (vestibular and cochlear)
   b. Nephrotoxicity
   c. Neurotoxicity (parasthesias, neuromuscular weakness)
4. Interactions
   a. Inactivation if administered with penicillins
   b. Additive ototoxicity with other aminoglycosides and loop diuretics
   c. Increased risk of nephrotoxicity with cephalosporins
   d. Possible respiratory paralysis with some inhalation anesthetics and neuromuscular blocking agents
5. Nursing implications
   a. Assess eighth cranial nerve function frequently for vertigo and hearing loss, usually of high frequencies. Permanent damage may occur without immediate intervention
   b. Monitor renal function for nephrotoxicity
   c. Monitor serum peak and trough drug levels
   d. Maintain hydration at 1,500 to 2,000 ml/day
6. Drug examples
   a. Amikacin (Amikin)
   b. Kanamycin (Kantrex)
   c. Gentamicin (Garamycin)
   d. Neomycin (Neo-IM)

      e. Netilmicin (Netromycin)
      f. Streptomycin (Strycin)
      g. Tobramycin (Nebcin)

E. Tetracyclines: specific information
1. Indications: active against some gram-positive and some gram-negative organisms, although many are resistant. Commonly used to treat unusual organisms *(Mycoplasma, Chlamydia, Rickettsia)*, gonorrhea and syphilis in penicillin-allergic patients, and acne. Demeclocycline is also used as a diuretic for treatment of syndrome of inappropriate ADH (SIADH)
2. Contraindications: during pregnancy and in children under age 8; may cause permanent staining of teeth
3. Side effects
    a. GI upset, hepatotoxicity, pancreatitis
    b. Photosensitivity, rash
    c. Pain at I.M. site, phlebitis at I.V. site
4. Interactions
    a. Decreased absorption results if taken with calcium supplements, iron, antacids, and magnesium-containing laxatives
    b. Tetracycline may increase the effects of oral anticoagulants
    c. Milk or dairy products decrease absorption of tetracycline
5. Nursing implications: Use glucose oxidase reagent (Clinistix or Tes-Tape) to test urine glucose; may cause false positive urine glucose results when tested with copper sulfate method (Clinitest)
6. Patient teaching
    a. Advise patient to avoid taking calcium supplements, antacids, magnesium-containing laxatives, iron supplements, and milk or dairy products (tetracycline) within 1 to 3 hours of these drugs
    b. Tell patient to use sunscreen and protective clothing to prevent photosensitivity reactions
    c. Caution patient to discard outdated or decomposed tetracyclines because they may be toxic
    d. Tell patient that these drugs may cause staining of soft contact lenses
7. Drug examples
    a. Tetracycline (Achromycin)
    b. Demeclocycline (Declomycin)
    c. Doxycycline (Vibramycin)
    d. Minocycline (Minocin)
    e. Oxytetracycline (Terramycin)

F. Miscellaneous anti-infectives: specific information
1. Indications
    a. Penicillin-resistant staphylococci (vancomycin)
    b. Anaerobic organisms, including *Bacteroides* and *Trichomonas vaginalis* (metronidazole)

   2. Side effects
      a. GI upset, hepatotoxicity (erythromycin)
      b. Pseudomembranous colitis (clindamycin)
      c. Bone marrow depression (chloramphenicol)
      d. Ototoxicity, nephrotoxicity (vancomycin)
   3. Interactions
      a. Additive ototoxicity and nephrotoxicity occur with other ototoxic and nephrotoxic drugs (vancomycin)
      b. Use with alcohol may cause a disulfiram-like reaction, nausea, vomiting, tachycardia, flushing, sweating. May also prolong bleeding with warfarin (metronidazole)
   4. Drug examples
      a. Chloramphenicol (Chloromycetin)
      b. Clindamycin (Cleocin)
      c. Erythromycin (E-mycin, Erythrocin)
      d. Metronidazole (Flagyl)
      e. Vancomycin (Vancocin)

Points to Remember

Antibacterials kill or inhibit the growth of susceptible bacteria.

Antibiotics (antibacterials) may affect a limited variety of bacteria (narrow spectrum) or a wide variety of bacteria (broad spectrum).

Specimens for culture and sensitivity should be taken before initiating therapy with antibacterials, but the first dose may be administered before receiving the results.

Patient education should emphasize the importance of compliance with the full course of therapy, even if the patient feels better. The patient should also be told that sharing antibacterials may be dangerous.

Inadequate antibacterial therapy—caused by too short a course, stopping the course prematurely, or too low a dose—may lead to exacerbations of the infection and the development of resistant organisms.

Glossary

Cross-sensitivity—hypersensitivity or allergy to one anti-infective in a group (for example, penicillins) that may result in an allergic reaction to another anti-infective in the same group

Gram-negative—having the pink color of counterstain used in Gram's method of staining microorganisms

Gram-positive—having the violet color of stain used in Gram's method of staining microorganisms; named after Hans Gram, Danish physician

Peak and trough drug concentration levels—serum drug concentration levels measured to determine whether the dosing regimen is therapeutic and to prevent toxicity. The peak concentration level is drawn immediately after the I.V. infusion of the drug. The trough concentration level is drawn just before administering the next dose

Superinfection—a new infection caused by an organism that is usually resistant to the anti-infective used to treat the initial infection. Signs of superinfection include furry overgrowth on the tongue, loose or foul-smelling stools, and vaginal itching or discharge

The Patient with a Urinary Tract Infection

Learning Objectives

After studying this section, the reader should be able to:

- Identify the nursing implications during assessment, implementation, and evaluation of the patient receiving drugs to treat a urinary tract infection.

- Discuss appropriate patient teaching for the patient receiving drugs to treat a urinary tract infection.

- Give examples of drugs used to treat urinary tract infections.

- Explain the indications for use of the sulfonamides.

- List the common side effects of drugs used to treat urinary tract infections.

XXIX. The Patient with a Urinary Tract Infection

A. Urinary tract drugs: general information

1. Mechanism of action: highly concentrated in the urine and provide a local antibacterial effect within the urinary tract
2. Indications: infections caused by susceptible organisms; use may be limited in systemic infections due to resistance or low concentrations in serum
3. Contraindications: hypersensitivity
4. Side effects: see specific information
5. Interactions: see specific information
6. Nursing implications
   a. Assessment: assess patient for signs and symptoms of urinary tract infection (frequency, urgency and burning on urination, flank pain). Obtain specimens for culture and sensitivity before administration
   b. Implementation: maintain a hydration of 2,000 to 3,000 ml/day to minimize crystalluria
   c. Evaluation: base on resolution of the signs and symptoms of urinary tract infection
7. Patient teaching: instruct patient to take these drugs around the clock

B. Sulfonamides: specific information

1. Indications
   a. Urinary tract infections (sulfamethoxazole, sulfisoxazole, sulfamethoxazole/trimethoprim)
   b. Ulcerative colitis (sulfasalazine)
   c. Conjunctivitis (sulfacetamide)
   d. *Pneumocystis carinii* pneumonia (sulfamethoxazole/trimethoprim)
   e. Bacterial infections, for example, otitis media, (sulfamethoxazole/trimethoprim)
2. Contraindications: pregnancy, lactation, hypersensitivity to sulfa drugs
3. Side effects
   a. Blood dyscrasias (for example, agranulocytosis, aplastic anemia)
   b. Rash, photosensitivity
   c. Crystalluria
   d. Nausea, vomiting, fever
4. Interactions: may increase hypoglycemic effects of oral hypoglycemics
5. Patient teaching
   a. Tell patient to use sunscreen and protective clothing to prevent photosensitivity reactions
   b. Inform patient that sulfasalazine may turn skin and urine a yellow-orange color, which is medically insignificant
   c. Instruct patient taking sulfacetamide on correct technique for instillation of eye drops and ointment
6. Drug examples
   a. Sulfamethoxazole (Gantanol, Urobak)
   b. Sulfamethoxazole/trimethoprim (Bactrim, Septra)

    c. Sulfisoxazole (Gantrisin, Lipo-Gantrisin)
    d. Sulfasalazine (Azaline, Azulfidine)
    e. Sulfacetamide (Bleph, Isopto Cetamide, Sulamyd)

C. Miscellaneous urinary tract medications: specific information
  1. Indications
    a. Treatment and prophylaxis of urinary tract infections (methenamine, nalidixic acid, nitrofurantoin)
    b. Urinary tract analgesic (phenazopyridine)
  2. Side effects
    a. GI upset, hypersensitivity
    b. Photosensitivity, peripheral neuropathy (nitrofurantoin)
    c. Blood dyscrasias (nalidixic acid, nitrofurantoin)
  3. Patient teaching: inform patient that nitrofurantoin may turn urine rust-yellow and phenazopyridine may turn urine red-orange
  4. Drug examples
    a. Methenamine (Mandelamine, Hiprex)
    b. Nalidixic acid (NegGram)
    c. Nitrofurantoin (Furadantin, Macrodantin)
    d. Phenazopyridine (Pyridium)

Points to Remember

Urinary tract infections are treated with antibacterials (antibiotics).

The signs and symptoms of urinary tract infections include frequency and urgency of urination, burning on urination, and flank pain.

Medications for urinary tract infections should be taken around the clock.

The sulfonamides are also used to treat ulcerative colitis, conjunctivitis, and *Pneumocystis carinii* pneumonia.

Glossary

Dyscrasia—disease

Pneumocystis carinii pneumonia—pneumonia caused by a parasite; formerly seen only in cancer and transplant patients taking immunosuppressants; now the leading cause of death in patients with acquired immune deficiency syndrome (AIDS)

Prophylaxis—prevention of disease

Ulcerative colitis—chronic, inflammatory disease of the large intestine, characterized by recurrent ulceration

The Patient with a Fungal Infection

Learning Objectives

After studying this section, the reader should be able to:

- Describe the mechanism of action of antifungal drugs.

- Identify the nursing implications during assessment, implementation, and evaluation of the patient receiving antifungal drugs.

- Discuss appropriate patient teaching for the patient receiving antifungal drugs.

- List the common side effects of antifungal drugs.

XXX. The Patient with a Fungal Infection

A. Antifungals: general information

1. Mechanism of action: kill or inhibit growth of fungi by inhibiting protein synthesis within the fungal cell or affecting the permeability of the fungal cell membrane
2. Indications: to treat fungal infections
3. Contraindications: hypersensitivity
4. Side effects: see specific information
5. Interactions: see specific information
6. Nursing implications
    a. Assessment: assess infected areas throughout therapy
    b. Implementation: obtain specimens for culture and sensitivity before administration. Wear gloves when applying topical preparations
    c. Evaluation: base on resolution of signs and symptoms of infection. Therapy may require weeks to months
7. Patient teaching
    a. Instruct patient on correct technique for vaginal application of tablets. Sanitary napkins may prevent staining of clothing. Patients should continue use during menstruation. During vaginal infections, sexual contact should be avoided or the partner should wear a condom to prevent reinfection
    b. Tell patient that occlusive dressings should not be used with topical preparations unless specifically ordered by physician
    c. Emphasize the importance of compliance with the therapeutic regimen

B. Antifungals: specific information

1. Indications
    a. Serious systemic fungal infections (amphotericin B, flucytosine)
    b. Oral and vaginal *Candida* infections (clotrimazole, miconazole, nystatin)
    c. Tinea (ringworm) infections (griseofulvin)
    d. Pulmonary, systemic, and subcutaneous fungal infections (ketoconazole)
2. Side effects
    a. Nausea, vomiting (amphotericin B, clotrimazole, flucytosine, ketoconazole, oral nystatin)
    b. Headache, hypotension, hypokalemia, fever, chills, dyscrasias, phlebitis, nephrotoxicity (amphotericin B)
    c. Blood dyscrasias (amphotericin B, flucytosine)
    d. Pruritus, skin irritation (miconazole)
    e. Photosensitivity (griseofulvin)
3. Interactions
    a. Additive nephrotoxicity occurs with other nephrotoxic agents
    b. Diuretics may potentiate hypokalemia (amphotericin B)

       c. Additive bone marrow depression occurs with similar-acting drugs (flucytosine)

       d. Alcohol may cause tachycardia, flushing, and added central nervous sytem depression if taken with griseofulvin and increased hepatotoxicity if taken with ketoconazole

       e. The effects of oral anticoagulants may be decreased with griseofulvin and increased with ketoconazole

4. Nursing implications: amphotericin B should be administered to hospitalized patients or those under close medical supervision. Monitor closely for 1 to 2 hours after each dose for fever, chills, nausea, vomiting, headache, and phlebitis. Administer via infusion pump for accurate rate

5. Patient teaching: tell patient taking griseofulvin to use sunscreen and protective clothing to prevent photosensitivity reactions

6. Drug examples

       a. Amphotericin B (Fungizone)

       b. Clotrimazole (Lotrimin, Mycelex)

       c. Griseofulvin (Fulvicin P/G or U/F, Grifulvin V, Grisactin)

       d. Flucytosine (5-FC, Ancoban)

       e. Ketoconazole (Nizoral)

       f. Miconazole (Micatin, Monistat)

       g. Nystatin (Mycostatin)

Points to Remember

Antifungals kill or inhibit the growth of fungi by inhibiting protein synthesis within the fungal cell or affecting the permeability of the fungal cell membrane.

Gloves should be warn when applying topical preparations to prevent spread of infection.

The patient should be aware that therapy for a fungal infection could take weeks or months.

Amphotericin B should be administered via an infusion pump to ensure an accurate rate.

Glossary

Hypokalemia—abnormally low amount of potassium in bloodstream, characterized by muscular weakness, tetany, orthostatic hypotension

Nephrotoxicity—the quality of being toxic to or capable of destruction of kidney cells

Phlebitis—vein inflammation

Pruritus—itching

The Patient with a Viral Infection

Learning Objectives

After studying this section, the reader should be able to:

- Describe the mechanism of action of antiviral drugs.

- Identify the nursing implications during assessment, implementation, and evaluation of the patient receiving antiviral drugs.

- List the common side effects of antiviral drugs.

- Discuss appropriate patient teaching for the patient receiving antiviral drugs.

XXXI. The Patient with a Viral Infection

A. Antivirals: general information
1. Mechanism of action
   a. Inhibit viral replication (acyclovir, vidarabine)
   b. Prevent penetration of the virus into host cells (amantadine)
2. Indications: susceptible viral infections
3. Contraindications: hypersensitivity
4. Side effects: see specific information
5. Interactions: see specific information
6. Nursing implications
   a. Assessment: assess lesions daily during therapy
   b. Evaluation: base on resolution of signs and symptoms of infection, crusting over of skin lesions, reepithelialization of cornea in herpes keratitis, improved neurologic status in herpetic encephalitis, and prevention of influenza A viral infections
7. Patient teaching: see specific information

B. Antiviral agents: specific information
1. Indications
   a. Genital herpes simplex (acyclovir)
   b. Herpes simplex encephalitis and keratitis (vidarabine)
   c. Prevention of influenza A viral infections (amantadine)
   d. Ophthalmic herpes simplex (trifluridine)
2. Side effects
   a. Dizziness, ataxia, headache (acyclovir, amantadine)
   b. Diarrhea, nausea, vomiting (acyclovir, vidarabine)
   c. Phlebitis at I.V. site (acyclovir, vidarabine)
   d. Renal failure (acyclovir)
   e. Hypotension (amantadine)
3. Interactions
   a. Probenecid increases blood levels of acyclovir
   b. Additive nephrotoxicity occurs with similar-acting drugs (acyclovir)
   c. Allopurinol may increase risk of side effects (vidarabine)
   d. Additive anticholinergic effects occurs with similar-acting drugs (amantadine)
4. Nursing implications
   a. Maintain adequate hydration in patients on acyclovir to prevent crystalluria
   b. Administer I.V. infusions via infusion pump to ensure accurate dose
5. Patient teaching
   a. Instruct patient on correct technique for topical or ophthalmic application.

      b. Advise patient that gloves should be used for topical preparations to prevent spread of infection

      c. Caution patient with skin lesions that over-the-counter preparations may delay healing

      d. Advise patient with genital herpes simplex that acyclovir is not a cure and will not prevent the spread of infection to others.

      e. Advise patient to abstain from sexual contact while lesions are present; condoms should be worn during all sexual contact

6. Drug examples

      a. Acyclovir (Zorivax)

      b. Vidarabine (Vira-A)

      c. Amantadine (Symmetrel)

      d. Trifluridine (Viroptic)

Points to Remember

Antiviral drugs either inhibit viral replication or prevent viral penetration into the host cell.

Intravenous antivirals should be administered via an infusion pump to ensure an accurate rate.

Gloves should be worn when applying topical preparations to prevent spread of infection.

The patient with genital herpes simplex should be aware that acyclovir is not a cure and will not prevent spread of infection.

Glossary

Herpes keratitis—infection of cornea by herpes simplex virus, leading to chronic inflammation, scarring, and possible vision loss

Herpetic encephalitis—acute brain disease caused by herpes simplex virus, characterized by early, repeated seizures and signs indicating temporal or frontal lobe involvement

Host cell—cell in which a parasitic organism is nourished and harbored

Virus—microorganism that can only reproduce inside the cells of a plant or animal host

The Patient with Tuberculosis

Learning Objectives

After studying this section, the reader should be able to:

- Describe the mechanism of action of antitubercular agents.

- List common side effects of antitubercular agents.

- Identify the nursing implications during assessment, implementation, and evaluation of the patient receiving antitubercular agents.

- Discuss appropriate patient teaching for the patient receiving antitubercular agents.

XXXII. The Patient with Tuberculosis

A. Antitubercular agents: general information

1. Mechanism of action: kill or inhibit the growth of *Mycobacterium* responsible for causing tuberculosis
2. Indications: to prevent or treat tuberculosis
3. Contraindications: hypersensitivity and severe liver disease
4. Side effects: nausea, vomiting, hepatitis
5. Interactions: alcohol may increase the risk of hepatotoxicity
6. Nursing implications
    a. Assessment: assess lung sounds, character and amount of sputum
    b. Implementation: obtain specimens for culture and sensitivity before initiating therapy
    c. Evaluation: base on diminished cough and sputum production, decreased fever and night sweats, reduced fatigue
7. Patient teaching
    a. Emphasize the importance of compliance with therapy, even if feeling well. Therapy may continue for 1 to 2 years
    b. Tell patient to avoid alcohol while taking these drugs

B. Antitubercular agents: specific information

1. Side effects
    a. Peripheral neuropathy (isoniazid)
    b. Abdominal cramps, diarrhea, headache, ataxia (rifampin)
    c. Optic neuritis (ethambutol)
    d. Neurotoxicity, vitamin B_{12} and folic acid deficiency (cycloserine)
    e. Nephrotoxicity, ototoxicity (streptomycin)
2. Interactions
    a. Antacids delay the absorption of isoniazid
    b. Isoniazid may cause additive central nervous system toxicity with other antituberculars
    c. Isoniazid inhibits the metabolism of phenytoin
    d. Rifampin may decrease the effectiveness of narcotic analgesics, oral hypoglycemic agents, oral anticoagulants, estrogens, and oral contraceptives
3. Nursing implications
    a. Pyridoxine (vitamin B_6) may be given with isoniazid to decrease peripheral neuropathy
    b. The patient taking ethambutol should be assessed frequently for visual changes. Visual impairment may be permanent if not identified early
    c. Patients taking aminosalicylic acid should receive 2,000 to 3,000 ml/day of fluids to prevent crystalluria

4. Patient teaching
    a. Inform patient taking rifampin that it may color saliva, sputum, sweat, tears, urine, and feces red-orange to red-brown
    b. Inform patient taking rifampin that it may permanently discolor soft contact lenses
    c. Tell patient taking rifampin to use a nonhormonal form of contraception
5. Drug examples
    a. Isoniazid (INH, Laniazid, Nydrazid)
    b. Rifampin (Rifadin, Rimactane)
    c. Ethambutol (Myambutol)
    d. Cycloserine (Seromycin)
    e. Streptomycin

Points to Remember

Antitubercular agents are used to prevent or treat tuberculosis.

The patient should understand that drug therapy for tuberculosis may continue for 1 to 2 years.

Vitamin B_6 can be given with isoniazid to decrease peripheral neuropathy.

The patient taking ethambutol should be assessed frequently for visual changes because visual impairment may be permanent if not identified early.

Glossary

Crystalluria—presence of crystals in urine

Hepatotoxicity—the quality of being toxic to or capable of destruction of liver cells

Optic neuritis—inflammation, and usually degeneration, of optic nerve

Peripheral neuropathy—inflammation and degeneration of peripheral nerves

The Patient with a Musculoskeletal Disorder

Learning Objectives

After studying this section, the reader should be able to:

● Describe the mechanism of action of the antigout agents, anti-inflammatory agents, and skeletal muscle relaxants.

● List the indications for the use of each of these drug classes.

● Describe the common side effects for each of these drug classes.

● Identify the nursing implications during assessment, implementation, and evaluation of the patient receiving each of these drug classes.

● Discuss appropriate patient teaching for the patient receiving each of these drug classes.

XXXIII. The Patient with a Musculoskeletal Disorder

A. Drugs for musculoskeletal disorders: general information
1. Mechanism of action
    a. Antigout agents use varying mechanisms to prevent or relieve gout
    b. Agents used to treat arthritis decrease the inflammatory process
    c. Skeletal muscle relaxants act centrally or directly to prevent or relieve muscle spasm
2. Indications: see specific information
3. Contraindications and precautions
    a. Antigout agents should be used cautiously in GI, renal, or hepatic disease
    b. Gold compounds are contraindicated in severe renal or hepatic dysfunction, uncontrolled diabetes mellitus, congestive heart failure, systemic lupus erythematosus, or recent radiation therapy
    c. Baclofen and oral dantrolene should not be given to the patient who uses spasticity to maintain posture and balance
4. Interactions: see specific information
5. Side effects: see specific information
6. Nursing implications
    a. Assessment: assess involved joints for pain, mobility, and edema
    b. Evaluation: base on improved mobility and decreased pain and edema
7. Patient teaching: see specific information

B. Antigout agents: specific information
1. Mechanism of action
    a. Reduce the inflammatory process (colchicine)
    b. Decrease production of uric acid (allopurinol)
    c. Enhance renal excretion of uric acid (probenecid, sulfinpyrazone)
2. Indications
    a. To treat active gout (colchicine)
    b. To prevent recurrent attacks of gout (allopurinol, probenecid)
3. Side effects
    a. Nausea, vomiting, diarrhea
    b. Bone marrow depression
    c. Rash (allopurinol, probenecid)
    d. Headache, uric acid kidney stones (probenecid, sulfinpyrazone)
4. Interactions
    a. Probenecid and sulfinpyrazone may cause higher and longer-sustained blood levels of many drugs
    b. Allopurinol increases toxicity of 6-mercaptopurine and azathioprine and increases the effects of oral hypoglycemics and the half-life of anticoagulants
    c. Aspirin may elevate uric acid levels
5. Nursing implications: fluid intake of at least 2,000 to 3,000 ml/day is necessary to prevent kidney stone formation

6. Patient teaching
   a. Emphasize the importance of compliance with therapy. Irregular administration may cause elevated uric acid levels and precipitate an attack of gout
   b. Instruct patient to follow physician's recommendations regarding weight loss, diet, and consumption of alcohol
   c. Caution against taking aspirin with these drugs
7. Drug examples
   a. Colchicine
   b. Allopurinol (Zyloprim, Lopurin)
   c. Probenecid (Benemid)
   d. Sulfinpyrazone (Anturane)

C. Arthritis preparations: specific information

1. Indications: treatment of arthritis is initiated with salicylates and nonsteroidal anti-inflammatory agents (see Section II). Rheumatoid arthritis resistant to these drugs may be treated with glucocorticoids (see Section XXIII) or gold compounds
2. Side effects: gold compounds
   a. Dizziness, rash, dermatitis, photosensitivity
   b. Metallic taste, stomatitis, diarrhea, abdominal pain
   c. Thrombocytopenia, aplastic anemia, agranulocytosis
3. Interactions: gold compounds may cause additive bone marrow depression with agents with similar side effects
4. Nursing implications
   a. Concurrent therapy with salicylates, nonsteroidal anti-inflammatory agents, or glucocorticoids is usually necessary, especially during the first few months of therapy
   b. Symptoms of toxicity include pruritus, skin rash, metallic taste, stomatitis, and diarrhea. If toxicity occurs, dimercaprol (BAL) may be given to enhance gold excretion
5. Patient teaching
   a. Advise patient to report signs of toxicity promptly
   b. Emphasize the necessity of good oral hygiene to prevent stomatitis
   c. Instruct patient to use sunscreen and protective clothing to prevent photosensitivity reactions
6. Drug examples
   a. Auranofin (Ridaura)
   b. Aurothioglucose (Solganal)
   c. Sodium gold thiomalate, aurothiomalate (Myochrysine)

D. Skeletal muscle relaxants: specific information

1. Mechanism of action
   a. Centrally acting (baclofen, carisoprodol, cyclobenzaprine, diazepam, methocarbamol)
   b. Direct-acting (dantrolene)

2. Indications
   a. Spasticity associated with spinal cord diseases or lesions (baclofen, dantrolene)
   b. Adjunctive therapy in acute painful musculoskeletal conditions (carisoprodol, cyclobenzaprine, diazepam, methocarbamol)
   c. Prevention and treatment of malignant hyperthermia (dantrolene)
3. Side effects
   a. Dizziness, drowsiness
   b. Nausea, GI upset
   c. Physical and psychological dependency (diazepam)
4. Interactions
   a. Additive CNS depression occurs with other CNS depressants and alcohol
   b. Use with monoamine oxidase (MAO) inhibitors may lead to hypertensive crisis and death (baclofen, cyclobenzaprine)
   c. Additive anticholinergic effects occur with antihistamines and antidepressants (cyclobenzaprine)
5. Patient teaching
   a. Caution patient to avoid activities requiring alertness until effects of drugs are known
   b. Tell patient to avoid use of alcohol or CNS depressants while taking these drugs
6. Drug examples
   a. Baclofen (Lioresal)
   b. Carisoprodol (Soma, Rela)
   c. Cyclobenzaprine (Flexeril)
   d. Dantrolene (Dantrium)
   e. Diazepam (Valium)
   f. Methocarbamol (Robaxin)

Points to Remember

Antigout agents work by decreasing inflammation, decreasing uric acid production, and increasing uric acid excretion.

The toxic side effects of gold compounds (pruritus, skin rash, metallic taste, stomatitis, diarrhea, bone marrow suppression) limit their use in the treatment of rheumatoid arthritis to patients unresponsive to treatment with aspirin, glucocorticoids, and nonsteroidal anti-inflammatory agents.

Skeletal muscle relaxants are used to treat spasticity with spinal cord diseases or lesions and as adjunctive therapy in acute painful musculoskeletal conditions.

Skeletal muscle relaxants work directly by acting on the neuromuscular junction or indirectly by acting on the central nervous system.

Glossary

Gout—a disorder of purine metabolism causing high serum levels of uric acid that results in pain and inflammation of the joints, usually beginning in the knee or foot

Malignant hyperthermia—a potentially fatal reaction to inhalation anesthetics characterized by a marked increase in the rate of muscle metabolism, a rapid rise in temperature, and muscular rigidity

Spasticity—increased tone or contractions of muscles caused by an upper motor neuron lesion that results in stiff, awkward movements

Uric acid—acid crystals produced from purine metabolism

The Patient with a Neoplastic Disorder

Learning Objectives

After studying this section, the reader should be able to:

● Explain the rationale for use of antineoplastic agents in the treatment of cancer.

● List the major side effects of the antineoplastic agents.

● Identify the nursing implications during assessment, implementation, and evaluation of the patient receiving an antineoplastic agent.

● Describe precautions for self-protection that the nurse must take when administering antineoplastic agents.

● Discuss appropriate patient teaching for the patient receiving an antineoplastic agent.

XXXIV. The Patient with a Neoplastic Disorder

A. Antineoplastic agents: general information

1. Mechanism of action: kill or inhibit reproduction of cancer cells. Action may not be limited to neoplastic cells. Cell cycle specific agents affect cells that are in only a certain phase of reproductive cycle. Cell cycle nonspecific agents affect cells regardless of phase in reproductive cycle

2. Indications: used to treat various solid tumors, lymphomas, and leukemias Usually used in combination to increase response and minimize toxicity Chemotherapy may be combined with other modalities such as surgery and radiation

3. Contraindications and precautions
   a. Neoplastic drugs are contraindicated in previous bone marrow depression, pregnancy, and lactation
   b. Their use requires caution in patients with decreased bone marrow reserve, radiation therapy, infections, and in patients who could become pregnant

4. Side effects
   a. Bone marrow depression: thrombocytopenia, leukemia, anemia
   b. Nausea, vomiting

5. Interactions: additive bone marrow depression

6. Nursing implications
   a. Assessment: monitor complete blood count, differential, and platelet count. Assess patient for nausea and vomiting during administration; antiemetics may be needed. Many I.V. agents are irritating to veins; monitor for phlebitis. Extravasation may cause tissue necrosis; follow protocol for treatment
   b. Implementation: prepare solutions for I.V. administration in a biologic cabinet. Gloves, gown, and mask should be worn while handling I.V. medications. Discard I.V. equipment in designated containers, according to protocol. Do not use I.M. injections or take temperature rectally. Give in short, high-dose, intermittent courses to maximize antineoplastic effects while allowing for recovery of normal cells. Maintain fluid intake of at least 2,000 ml/day
   c. Evaluation: base on decrease in size and spread of cancer without toxic side effects

7. Patient teaching
   a. Tell patient to notify physician immediately if fever, sore throat, signs of infection, or unusual bleeding occur
   b. Tell patient to avoid crowds and persons with infections
   c. Instruct patient to use a soft toothbrush and an electric razor
   d. Instruct patient to avoid alcohol and aspirin-containing products
   e. Explain that patient should not receive vaccinations without consulting physician
   f. Discuss possibility of hair loss and ways to cope with this problem with patient taking agents causing alopecia

g. Discuss the need for contraception and the effects on fertility because many agents have teratogenic effects

h. Instruct patient at risk for stomatitis to inspect oral mucosa for erythema and ulceration, using a sponge brush, and to rinse mouth after meals if this occurs

B. Alkylating agents: specific information
1. Mechanism of action: alkylating agents affect DNA synthesis by cross-linking of DNA to inhibit reproduction. Cell cycle nonspecific
2. Side effects
   a. Alopecia (cyclophosphamide)
   b. Gonadal suppression (chlorambucil, cyclophosphamide, mechlorethamine)
   c. Hyperuricemia (busulfan, chlorambucil, mechlorethamine)
   d. Ototoxicity, tinnitus, hypomagnesemia, hypokalemia, hypocalcemia, nephrotoxicity (cisplatin)
   e. Hemorrhagic cystitis, hematuria (cyclophosphamide)
3. Interactions
   a. Additive ototoxicity and nephrotoxicity occur with other ototoxic and nephrotoxic agents
   b. Phenobarbital may increase the effects of cyclophosphamide
4. Nursing implications: frequently assess patient taking cisplatin for dizziness, tinnitus, hearing loss, loss of coordination, and numbness or tingling of extremities; may be irreversible
5. Drug examples
   a. Busulfan (Myleran)
   b. Chlorambucil (Leukeran)
   c. Cisplatin (Platinol)
   d. Cyclophosphamide (Cytoxan, Neosar)
   e. Mechlorethamine (nitrogen mustard, Mustargen)

C. Antitumor antibiotics: specific information
1. Mechanism of action: antitumor antibiotics interfere with DNA and RNA synthesis. Cell cycle nonspecific
2. Side effects
   a. Alopecia, stomatitis, phlebitis at I.V. site, gonadal suppression, hyperuricemia
   b. Congestive heart failure, dysrhythmias (daunorubicin)
   c. Cardiomyopathy, EKG changes (doxorubicin)
3. Nursing implications
   a. Monitor vital signs frequently during administration
   b. Assess patient taking daunorubicin for congestive heart failure (dyspnea, rales, peripheral edema, weight gain)
   c. Assess patient taking doxorubicin for myocardial toxicity (dyspnea, dysrhythmias, hypotension, weight gain)

4. Drug examples
   a. Dactinomycin (Actinomycin-D, Cosmegen)
   b. Daunorubicin (Cerubidine)
   c. Doxorubicin (Adriamycin)
   d. Bleomycin (Blenoxane)

D. Antimetabolites: specific information
   1. Mechanism of action: antimetabolites take the place of normal proteins required for DNA synthesis. Cell cycle specific
   2. Side effects
      a. Alopecia (cytarabine, fluorouracil, methotrexate)
      b. Stomatitis (cytarabine, fluorouracil, methotrexate)
      c. Hyperuricemia (cytarabine, mercaptopurine, methotrexate)
      d. Diarrhea, phototoxicity (fluorouracil)
      e. Hepatotoxicity (cytarabine, mercaptopurine, methotrexate)
   3. Interactions
      a. Mercaptopurine and methotrexate have additive hepatotoxicity with other hepatotoxic agents
      b. Allopurinol decreases metabolism and increases the risk of toxicity with mercaptopurine
      c. Salicylates, oral hypoglycemic agents, phenytoin, phenylbutazone, tetracyclines, probenecid, and chloramphenicol increase the risk of toxicity with methotrexate
   4. Nursing implications
      a. Assess patients taking fluorouracil for cerebellar dysfunction (dizziness, weakness, ataxia)
      b. Assess patients taking fluorouracil for stomatitis and diarrhea. These symptoms may necessitate discontinuation
      c. Ensure that the patient taking high doses of methotrexate receives folinic acid or citrovrum factor (Leucovorin rescue) to prevent fatal toxicity
   5. Patient teaching: tell patient taking fluorouracil or methotrexate to use sunscreen and wear protective clothing to prevent photosensitivity reactions
   6. Drug examples
      1. Cytarabine (ARA-C, cytosine arabinoside, Cytosar-U)
      2. Fluorouracil (5-FU, Adrucil, Efudex, Fluoroplex)
      3. Mercaptopurine (6-MP, Purinethol)
      4. Methotrexate (amethopterin, Folex, Mexate)

E. Hormonal agents (see Section XXIV): specific information
   1. Mechanism of action: hormonal agents cause immunosuppression and block normal hormones in tumors that are sensitive
   2. Side effects
      a. Edema, hypercalcemia (diethylstilbestrol, tamoxifen, testosterone)
      b. Impotence, gynecomastia in males (diethylstilbestrol, testosterone)

3. Interactions
    a. Diethylstilbestrol and testosterone may alter the effects of oral anticoagulants, oral hypoglycemic agents, and insulins
    b. Tamoxifen decreases the effectiveness of concurrently administered estrogen
4. Patient teaching: patients taking tamoxifen may have severe bone pain, which may indicate drug effectiveness and will resolve over time. Pain may be controlled with analgesics
5. Drug examples
    1. Diethylstilbestrol (DES)
    2. Megestrol (Megace, Pallace)
    3. Tamoxifen (Nolvadex)
    4. Testosterone (Andro, Depo-Testosterone, Testex)
    5. Prednisone (Deltasone)

F. **Vinca alkaloids: specific information**
    1. Mechanism of action: vinca alkaloids prevent mitosis. Cell cycle specific
    2. Side effects
        a. Peripheral neuropathy, hyperuricemia
        b. Stomatitis, anorexia, constipation, phlebitis at I.V. site
        c. Alopecia
    3. Drug examples
        a. vinblastine (Velban)
        b. vincristine (Oncovin)

Points to Remember

Antineoplastic agents kill or inhibit reproduction of tumor cells. These agents may affect the cell only during a specific portion of the reproductive cycle (cell cycle specific) or may affect the cell regardless of the phase in its reproductive cycle (cell cycle nonspecific).

Side effects of the antineoplastic agents result from their effects on normal cells.

The primary side effects of the antineoplastic agents are bone marrow depression, nausea, vomiting, alopecia, stomatitis, and gonadal suppression.

Antineoplastic solutions for I.V. administration should be prepared in a biological cabinet. Gloves, gown, and mask should be worn while handling I.V. medications. I.V. equipment should be discarded in designated containers.

Patient teaching should include methods to prevent infection, bleeding, and stomatitis, discussion of contraception and psychological effects, and conditions that warrant notifying the physician.

Glossary

Alopecia—loss of hair

Bone marrow depression—hematologic toxicity causing a decrease in blood cell production that can result in thrombocytopenia, leukopenia, and/or anemia

Cross-linking—inactivation of DNA by the formation of bonds that cause abnormal base pairing

Gonadal suppression—decrease in the number and/or function of reproductive cells

Stomatitis—inflammation and potential ulceration of the mucous membranes of the mouth

The Patient Requiring Immunosuppression

Learning Objectives

After studying this section, the reader should be able to:

- Describe the mechanism of action of the various immunosuppressants.

- Explain the rationale for use of immunosuppressants for the patient with a transplant.

- List the major side effects of immunosuppressants.

- Identify the precautions necessary to protect the immunosuppressed patient from infection.

- Discuss appropriate patient teaching for the patient receiving immunosuppressants.

XXXV. The Patient Requiring Immunosuppression

A. **Immunosuppressants: general information**
1. Mechanism of action
   a. Azathioprine causes suppression of cell-mediated immunity and altered antibody formation
   b. Cyclosporine inhibits T lymphocyte proliferation and function
   c. Glucocorticoids inhibit the formation and migration of macrophages and leukocytes toward areas of inflammation
2. Indications: see specific information
3. Contraindications and precautions: contraindicated in pregnancy and lactation
4. Side effects: nausea, vomiting, diarrhea, anorexia, hepatotoxicity, leukopenia, anemia, thrombocytopenia
5. Interactions: see specific information
6. Nursing implications
   a. Assessment: assess patient for infection
   b. Implementation: protect transplant patients from staff and visitors with infections. Maintain protective isolation as indicated
   c. Evaluation: base on lack of rejection of transplanted tissues
7. Patient teaching
   a. Emphasize the need for compliance with life-long therapy to prevent transplant rejection
   b. Tell patient to report signs of infection, unusual bleeding, or transplant rejection immediately to physician
   c. Discuss the potential for teratogenic effects of these drugs during pregnancy and the need for contraception

B. **Immunosuppressants: specific information**
1. Indication
   a. To prevent rejection of renal transplants (azathioprine)
   b. To prevent rejection of renal, hepatic, and cardiac transplants (cyclosporine). Usually combined with glucocorticoids
   c. To treat rheumatoid arthritis unresponsive to conventional therapy (azathioprine)
2. Contraindications: azathioprine is used cautiously in patients with bone marrow depression, infections, and malignancies
3. Side effects
   a. Fever, chills (azathioprine)
   b. Tremor, hypertension, hirsutism, gingival hyperplasia, nephrotoxicity, infections (cyclosporine)
   c. Fragile skin, mood swings, peptic ulcer, edema, hirsutism, altered fat distribution, increased blood sugar

4. Interactions
   a. Additive myelosuppression occurs with azathioprine
   b. Allopurinol increases the risk of toxicity of azathioprine
   c. Cyclosporine has additive nephrotoxicity with other nephrotoxic drugs
   d. Ketoconazole and cimetidine increase the toxicity risk of cyclosporine
   e. Rifampin, phenobarbital, phenytoin, and sulfamethoxazole-trimethoprim I.V. decrease the effects of cyclosporine
5. Nursing implications: monitor serum cyclosporine levels. Monitor intake and output; decrease in urine output may lead to toxicity of azathioprine
6. Patient teaching: instruct patient taking cyclosporine to maintain good oral hygiene to prevent gingival hyperplasia
7. Drug examples
   a. Azathioprine (Imuran)
   b. Cyclosporine (Sandimmune)
   c. Prednisone (Deltasone)

Points to Remember

Immunosuppressants are used to prevent rejection of transplants.

Immunosuppressed patients must be protected from and monitored for infection.

Patient teaching should emphasize the importance of compliance with the therapeutic regimen. Immunosuppressive therapy is life-long for patients with transplants.

Patients should be taught to report signs of infection, unusual bleeding, or transplant rejection immediately to the physician.

Glossary

Cell-mediated immunity—the production of lymphocytes by the thymus in response to exposure to antigens, such as those in tissue transplantation

Myelosuppression—inhibition of bone marrow function

Rejection—destruction of transplanted material at the cellular level by the host's immune response

Teratogenic effects—the development of abnormal structures in an embryo resulting in fetal deformity

T lymphocytes—lymphocytic cells that develop in the thymus and become the initiators of cellular immune response

The Patient with Gastric Hyperacidity

Learning Objectives

After studying this section, the reader should be able to:

● Describe the mechanism of action of antacids and histamine antagonists.

● List the major side effects of antacids and histamine antagonists.

● Identify the nursing implications during assessment, implementation, and evaluation of the patient receiving antacids or histamine antagonists.

● Discuss appropriate patient teaching for the patient receiving antacids or histamine antagonists.

XXXVI. The Patient with Gastric Hyperacidity

A. Drugs for gastric hyperacidity: general information

1. Mechanism of action
   a. Antacids partially neutralize gastric acid
   b. Histamine antagonists inhibit gastric acid secretion by inhibiting the action of histamine at the H_2 receptors in the gastric parietal cells
   c. Local-acting antiulcer agents act as a mucosal protectant by coating the ulcer crater
   d. Anticholinergics inhibit motility and gastric secretions
2. Indications: to prevent or treat peptic ulcer disease
3. Contraindications: see specific information
4. Side effects: see specific information
5. Interactions: see specific information
6. Nursing implications
   a. Assessment: assess patient for epigastric or abdominal pain and frank or occult bleeding
   b. Evaluation: base on decrease in abdominal pain, healing of ulcers on X-ray or endoscopy, or prevention of gastric irritation and bleeding
7. Patient teaching: tell patient to avoid alcohol, aspirin-containing products, and foods that cause GI irritation

B. Antacids: specific information

1. Indications
   a. Indigestion
   b. Reflux esophagitis
2. Contraindications and precautions
   a. Antacids are contraindicated in abdominal pain of unknown origin
   b. The use of magnesium-containing antacids requires caution in patients with renal failure
3. Side effects
   a. Constipation (aluminum), diarrhea (magnesium)
   b. Hypermagnesemia (magnesium), hypophosphatemia (aluminum)
4. Interactions
   a. Antacids decrease absorption of tetracycline, phenothiazines, iron, and isoniazid
   b. Large doses increase pH of urine
   c. Antacids cause premature dissolution of enteric coated tablets; separate by at least 1 hour
5. Nursing implications
   a. Antacids with aluminum and magnesium balance the laxative effects of magnesium and the constipating effects of aluminum
   b. Tablets must be chewed well and followed by half a glass of water

6. Patient teaching
   a. Instruct patient with congestive heart failure, hypertension, or on a sodium-restricted diet to check the drug label for sodium content and use low-sodium preparations
   b. Explain that antacids should not be taken for more than 2 weeks or for recurring problems without consulting a physician
7. Drug examples
   a. Aluminum hydroxide (Amphojel, ALternaGEL)
   b. Magaldrate (Riopan)
   c. Magnesium hydroxide and aluminum hydroxide (Gelusil, Maalox, Mylanta, WinGel)

C. **Histamine antagonists: specific information**
   1. Indications
      a. Active duodenal ulcer
      b. Gastric hypersecretory states (Zollinger-Ellison syndrome)
   2. Side effects: confusion, headache, dizziness
   3. Interactions
      a. Cimetidine may cause increased blood levels and toxicity of theophylline, metoprolol, propranolol, lidocaine, oral anticoagulants, quinidine, chlordiazepoxide, diazepam, and phenytoin
      b. Antacids may decrease the absorption of cimetidine and ranitidine
      c. Smoking may decrease the effectiveness of cimetidine and ranitidine
   4. Patient teaching: inform patient that smoking interferes with the actions of these drugs and should be avoided; if patient continues, he should at least avoid smoking after the last dose of the day
   5. Drug examples
      a. Cimetidine (Tagamet)
      b. Ranitidine (Zantac)

D. **Local acting antiulcer agents: specific information**
   1. Side effects: constipation
   2. Interactions
      a. These agents may decrease the absorption of cimetidine, phenytoin, warfarin, or tetracycline; separate by at least 2 hours
      b. Antacids may decrease effectiveness; separate by at least 1 hour
   3. Drug example: sucralfate (Carafate)

E. **Anticholinergic agents (see Section II): specific information**
   1. Indications: used as adjunctive therapy for peptic ulcer disease
   2. Side effects: tachycardia, dry mouth, constipation, urinary retention, urinary hesitancy
   3. Interactions
      a. Additive anticholinergic effects occur with similar-acting drugs
      b. Antacids may decrease the absorption of anticholinergics
   4. Drug examples
      a. Glycopyrrolate (Robinul)
      b. Propantheline (Pro-Banthine)

Points to Remember

Gastric hyperacidity is treated by neutralizing gastric acid, inhibiting acid secretions, or providing direct mucosal protection.

Histamine antagonists inhibit gastric acid secretion by inhibiting the action of histamine at the H_2 receptors in the gastric parietal cells.

The patient taking drugs for gastric hyperacidity should avoid alcohol, products containing aspirin, and foods that cause gastrointestinal irritation.

The patient should know that smoking may decrease the effectiveness of cimetidine and ranitidine, which are histamine antagonists.

Glossary

H_2 receptors—cells in the gastric mucosa that respond to the release of histamine by increasing the secretion of gastric acid

Motility—capable of spontaneous movement

Occult bleeding—blood not visible by gross inspection, that can be detected only by chemical methods (guaiac) or with a microscope

Peptic ulcer—lesion of mucous membrane of stomach, duodenum, or other part of the gastrointestinal system exposed to acid and pepsin gastric juices

The Patient Requiring Antiemetics or Emetics

Learning Objectives

After studying this section, the reader should be able to:

● Describe the mechanism of action of antiemetics and emetics.

● List common side effects of antiemetics and emetics.

● Identify the nursing implications during assessment, implementation, and evaluation of the patient receiving antiemetics or emetics.

● Discuss appropriate patient teaching for the patient receiving antiemetics or emetics.

XXXVII. The Patient Requiring Antiemetics or Emetics

A. **Antiemetics/emetics: general information**
1. Mechanism of action: see specific information
2. Indications: to prevent or treat nausea and vomiting (except ipecac)
3. Contraindications: see specific information
4. Side effects: drowsiness (except ipecac)
5. Interactions: antiemetics have additive central nervous system (CNS) depression with other CNS depressants, antihistamines, narcotics, and sedatives/hypnotics
6. Nursing implications: see specific information
7. Patient teaching: see specific information

B. **Antiemetics (see Section X): specific information**
1. Mechanism of action
    a. Act on chemoreceptor trigger zone to prevent nausea and vomiting (phenothiazines, trimethobenzamide, benzquinamide)
    b. Diminish motion sickness (dimenhydrinate, scopolamine, meclizine)
    c. Increase rate of gastric emptying (metoclopramide)
2. Contraindications
    a. Phenothiazines are contraindicated in narrow-angle glaucoma, bone marrow depression, or severe liver or cardiac disease
    b. Metoclopramide is contraindicated in patients with possible GI obstruction
3. Side effects
    a. Extrapyramidal reactions, photosensitivity, dry eyes, blurred vision, dry mouth, constipation (phenothiazines)
    b. Hypotension, pain at I.M. injection site, rectal irritation with suppositories (trimethobenzamide)
4. Interactions
    a. Additive hypotension occurs with other hypotensive agents (phenothiazines)
    b. Additive anticholinergic effects occur with anticholinergic drugs (phenothiazines and meclizine)
    c. Metoclopramide may affect the GI absorption of other drugs because of its effect on GI motility
5. Nursing implications
    a. Assessment: assess patient for nausea and vomiting
    b. Evaluation: base on prevention or relief of nausea and vomiting
6. Patient teaching
    a. Instruct patient taking phenothiazines to make position changes slowly to minimize orthostatic hypotension and to wear sunscreen and protective clothing to prevent photosensitivity reactions
    b. Caution patient to avoid activities requiring alertness until effects of the drug are known

    c. Explain that frequent mouth rinses, good oral hygiene, and sugarless gum or candy may minimize dry mouth

    d. Caution against concurrent use of alcohol

    e. Instruct patient in application of Transderm Scōp patches behind the ear at least 4 hours before exposure to motion sickness conditions. Oral drugs should be taken 1 hour before exposure

7. Drug examples

    a. Phenothiazines: perphenazine (Trilafon), prochlorperazine (Compazine), promazine (Sparine), promethazine (Phenergan), thiethylperazine (Torecan)

    b. Benzquinamide (Emete-con)

    c. Dimenhydrinate (Dramamine)

    d. Meclizine (Antivert, Bonine)

    e. Metoclopramide (Reglan)

    f. Scopolamine (Transderm Scōp)

    g. trimethobenzamide (Tigan)

C. Emetics: specific information

1. Mechanism of action: stimulate the chemoreceptor trigger zone in the central nervous system and gastric mucosa to induce vomiting

2. Indications: induction of vomiting in the early management of overdose and poisoning with noncaustic substances in conscious patients

3. Contraindications: contraindicated in semicomatose, inebriated, unconscious, or seizing patients or after ingestion of caustic substances

4. Side effects: dysrhythmias

5. Interactions: activated charcoal may reduce emetic effect

6. Nursing implications

    a. Assessment: assess level of consciousness before administration. Obtain a history to determine potential antidotes and if caustic substances were ingested

    b. Implementation: follow administration of syrup with one to two glasses of water. Fluid extract is 14 times more potent than syrup; do not confuse

    c. Evaluation: base on emesis within 30 minutes of administration

7. Patient teaching

    a. Instruct parents with children over age 1 to keep a small amount on hand for emergencies

    b. Instruct parents not to use this medication if caustic substances are ingested

8. Drug example: ipecac syrup

Points to Remember

Transderm Scōp patches should be applied behind the ear at least 4 hours before exposure to the condition expected to cause motion sickness.

Emetics are used in the treatment of poisoning or overdose when the substance is noncaustic and the patient is conscious.

Ipecac fluid extract is 14 times more potent than the syrup; they must not be confused.

Parents with children over age 1 should keep a small amount of ipecac syrup on hand for emergencies.

Glossary

Chemoreceptor trigger zone—the center in the medulla that controls vomiting

Emesis—vomiting

Orthostatic hypotension—abnormally low blood pressure that occurs when a person stands; also called postural hypotension

Photosensitivity—increased reaction of skin to sunlight; may result in edema, papules, urticara, or acute burns

The Patient with a Disorder of Intestinal Motility

Learning Objectives

After studying this section, the reader should be able to:

● Describe the mechanism of action of antidiarrheals and laxatives.

● List common side effects of antidiarrheals and laxatives.

● Identify the nursing implications during assessment, implementation, and evaluation of the patient receiving antidiarrheals or laxatives.

● Discuss appropriate patient teaching for the patient receiving antidiarrheals or laxatives.

● Explain how the mechanism of action for each type of laxative relates to its indication for use.

XXXVIII. The Patient with a Disorder of Intestinal Motility

A. Antidiarrheals/laxatives: general information

1. Mechanism of action: see specific information
2. Indications
    a. Antidiarrheals are used for the control and symptomatic relief of acute and chronic nonspecific diarrhea
    b. Laxatives are used to treat or prevent constipation or to prepare the bowel for radiologic or endoscopic procedures
3. Contraindications: contraindicated in persistent or severe abdominal pain of unknown etiology, especially when accompanied by fever
4. Side effects: see specific information
5. Interactions
    a. Kaolin may decrease the absorption of digoxin
    b. Laxatives may decrease the absorption of drugs taken orally by decreasing the transit time through the intestine
6. Nursing implications
    a. Assessment: assess the abdomen for pain, distention, and bowel sounds. Assess the frequency and consistency of stools
    b. Evaluation: base on production of soft, formed stool
7. Patient teaching: see specific information

B. Antidiarrheals: specific information

1. Mechanism of action
    a. Slow the intestinal motility (diphenoxylate/atropine, loperamide, paregoric)
    b. Decrease the fluid content of the stool (kaolin/pectin)
2. Side effects
    a. Constipation
    b. Drowsiness (diphenoxylate/atropine, loperamide, paregoric)
3. Interactions
    a. Additive central nervous system (CNS) depression with other CNS depressants (diphenoxylate/atropine, loperamide, paregoric)
    b. Additive anticholinergic properties with similar-acting drugs (diphenoxylate/atropine, loperamide)
4. Nursing implications
    a. Assess patient's skin turgor and fluid and electrolyte balance for dehydration
    b. Be aware that diphenoxylate/atropine has a potential for dependence with high-dose, long-term use. Atropine has been added to discourage abuse

      c. Do not confuse paregoric with deodorized tincture of opium, which is 25 times more potent

5. Patient teaching

      a. Caution patient to avoid activities requiring alertness until effects of drug are known (diphenoxylate/atropine, loperamide, paregoric)

      b. Tell patient to avoid alcohol and CNS depressants with these drugs (diphenoxylate/atropine, loperamide, paregoric)

      c. Tell patient to notify physician if diarrhea persists or fever occurs

6. Drug examples

      a. Bismuth subsalicylate (Pepto-Bismol)

      b. Diphenoxylate/atropine (Lomotil)

      c. Kaolin/pectin (Kaopectate)

      d. Loperamide (Imodium)

      e. Paregoric (camphorated tincture of opium)

C. Laxatives: specific information

1. Mechanism of action

      a. Bulk-forming agents absorb water into the fecal contents and expand, giving more bulk to the stool

      b. Lubricants retard water absorption from the stool and lubricate and soften intestinal contents

      c. Osmotic agents increase water content and soften the stool. Lactulose also inhibits the diffusion of ammonia from the colon into the blood

      d. Saline cathartics increase the bulk of intestinal contents and stimulate peristalsis

      e. Stimulant laxatives stimulate peristalsis and inhibit water and electrolyte reabsorption from the intestines

      f. Stool softeners allow more fluid and fat to penetrate feces, producing a softer fecal mass

2. Indications

      a. Psyllium (bulk-forming agent) may also be used in the management of chronic watery diarrhea

      b. Lactulose is used as an adjunct to manage hepatic encephalopathy

3. Side effects

      a. Nausea, vomiting, cramping

      b. Esophageal or intestinal obstruction (bulk-forming agents)

      c. Lipid pneumonia, nutritional deficiencies (lubricants)

      d. Cramps, distention, flatulence, belching (osmotic agents)

      e. Dehydration, electrolyte imbalance (saline cathartics)

4. Nursing implications

      a. Mix bulk-forming agents in a full glass of water or juice and give an additional glass of liquid after administration

      b. Assess the mental status of the patient being treated for hepatic encephalopathy

5. Patient teaching
   a. Encourage the patient to use other forms of bowel regulation (increasing bulk and fluid intake and exercise)
   b. Explain that most laxatives should be used for short-term therapy. Long-term therapy may cause electrolyte imbalance and dependence
6. Drug examples
   a. Bulk-forming agents: psyllium hydrophilic mucilloid (Effersyllium, Fiberall, Konsyl, Metamucil, Perdiem)
   b. Lubricants: mineral oil (Kondremul, Fleet Mineral Oil Enema)
   c. Osmotic agents: lactulose (Cephulac, Chronulac)
   d. Saline cathartics: magnesium citrate, magnesium hydroxide (Milk of Magnesia), magnesium sulfate (Epsom salts), phosphates/biphosphate (Fleet Phospho-soda)
   e. Stimulant: bisacodyl (Biscolax, Dulcolax), castor oil, cascara sagrada, glycerin suppositories, phenolphthalein (Ex-Lax), senna (Senokot)
   f. Stool softeners: docusate sodium sulfosuccinate (Colace, Docusate), dioctyl calcium sulfosuccinate (Surfak)

Points to Remember

Drugs affecting the digestive tract are contraindicated in abdominal pain of unknown etiology, especially if the patient is also febrile.

Laxatives should be used for short-term therapy. The patient should be encouraged to use other forms of bowel regulation, such as increasing bulk, fluid intake, and exercise.

Nursing assessment for the patient receiving digestive drugs includes the assessment of abdominal pain, distention, bowel sounds, frequency and consistency of stool, nausea and vomiting, and frank or occult bleeding.

Laxatives may decrease the absorption of drugs taken orally by decreasing the transit time through the intestine.

Glossary

Hepatic encephalopathy—changes in level of consciousness, mental status, behavior, and neurologic status caused by severe liver impairment

Intestinal obstruction—blockage of the lumen of the intestine

Lipid pneumonia—pneumonia after aspiration of oils, such as oily nosedrops or mineral oil

Skin turgor—normal resiliency of skin; dehydration causes decreased skin turgor characterized by lax skin which, when grasped, only slowly returns to position; edema causes increased turgor characterized by smooth, shiny skin that cannot be grasped

The Patient with an Eye Disorder

Learning Objectives

After studying this section, the reader should be able to:

- Explain the rationale for use of anti-infective agents, anti-inflammatory agents, anesthetics, lubricants, miotics, beta-adrenergic blocking agents, carbonic anhydrase inhibitors, osmotic agents, mydriatics, and cycloplegics for treating the patient with an eye disorder.

- Discuss appropriate patient teaching for the patient receiving medication for an eye disorder.

- Identify nursing implications during assessment, implementation, and evaluation of the patient receiving medication for an eye disorder.

- List common side effects of drugs used to treat eye disorders.

XXXIX. The Patient with an Eye Disorder

A. Drugs for eye disorders: general information
  1. Mechanism of action
      a. Anti-infective agents kill or inhibit growth of susceptible bacteria, fungi, and viruses
      b. Anti-inflammatory agents control inflammation and reduce the amount of loss of vision and scarring
      c. Anesthetics produce corneal anesthesia
      d. Lubricants replace tears or add moisture to the eye
      e. Miotics lower intraocular pressure by constricting the pupil, contracting the ciliary muscles, opening the anterior chamber angle, and increasing outflow
      f. Beta-adrenergic blocking agents lower intraocular pressure by decreasing sympathetic impulses to the eye and aqueous humor production. They do not affect accommodation or pupil size
      g. Carbonic anhydrase inhibitors decrease aqueous humor production
      h. Osmotic agents produce a profound diuresis that decreases intraocular pressure
      i. Mydriatics and cycloplegics dilate the pupil and paralyze accommodation
  2. Indications: see specific information
  3. Contraindications and precautions
      a. Anti-inflammatory agents are contraindicated in acute infections
      b. Miotics are contraindicated in secondary glaucoma, acute iritis, and inflammatory diseases
      c. Osmotic agents should be given cautiously to cardiac patients because they may precipitate congestive heart failure (CHF)
      d. Mydriatics are contraindicated in narrow-angle glaucoma
  4. Side effects: see specific information
  5. Interactions: none significant with local eye agents
  6. Nursing implications
      a. Assessment: assess patient for symptoms of eye disorder and possible side effects
      b. Implementation: wait at least 5 minutes before instilling a second eye medication. Eye medications always must be kept sterile
      c. Evaluation: base on resolution or control of symptoms of eye disorder
  7. Patient teaching
      a. Instruct patient on correct method for instilling eye medications
      b. Instruct patient with glaucoma to carry identification describing disorder and drug therapy

B. Anti-infective agents (see Section XXVIII): specific information
  1. Indications
      a. Antibacterials: susceptible ocular bacterial infections
      b. Antifungals: susceptible ocular fungal infections
      c. Antivirals: susceptible ocular viral infections

2. Side effects: superinfection, local irritation
3. Drug examples
   a. Antibacterials: bacitracin (Baciguent), chloramphenicol (Chloromycetin), erythromycin, gentamicin (Garamycin), kanamycin (Kantrex), lincomycin (Lincocin), neomycin (Myciguent), polymyxin B (Aerosporin), streptomycin, sulfisoxazole (Gantrisin)
   b. Antifungals: amphotericin B (Fungizone), nystatin (Mycostatin)
   c. Antivirals: idoxuridine (Herplex), vidarabine (Vira-A), trifluridine (Viroptic)

C. Anti-inflammatory agents (see Section XXIII): specific information
1. Indications: nonpyogenic inflammatory conditions of the eye
2. Side effects: cataracts, increased intraocular pressure, impaired healing, masking of infection
3. Drug examples
   a. Dexamethasone (Decadron)
   b. Hydrocortisone acetate (Cortril)
   c. Prednisolone acetate (Pred Forte)
   d. Dexamethasone and neomycin (Maxitrol)

D. Anesthetics: specific information
1. Indications: eye examinations and surgery
2. Side effects: temporary stinging or burning, temporary loss of corneal reflex
3. Nursing implications
   a. Eye anesthetics are used only for eye examinations and surgery and should not be given to the patient for home use
   b. An eye patch may be necessary to protect the eye from injury until the corneal reflex returns (about 1 hour)
4. Drug examples
   a. Proparacaine hydrochloride (Ophthaine)
   b. Tetracaine hydrochloride (Pontocaine)

E. Lubricants: specific information
1. Indications
   a. Replacement of tears
   b. Moistening of contact lenses or artificial eyes
   c. Keratitis
   d. Protection for eye during surgical or diagnostic procedures
2. Drug examples
   a. Methylcellulose (Cologel)
   b. Polyvinyl alcohol for hard contact lenses (Liquifilm Tears, Pre-Sert, Total, Tears Naturale)
   c. Petroleum-based ointments (Lacri-Lube)
   d. Hydroxypropyl cellulose (Lacriserts)

F. Miotics: specific information
1. Mechanism of action
   a. Cholinergics lower intraocular pressure by mimicking the action of acetylcholine
   b. Cholinesterase inhibitors lower intraocular pressure by inhibiting the action of cholinesterase
2. Indications: to lower intraocular pressure in open-angle glaucoma; topical medication
3. Side effects
   a. Ocular: myopia, decreased vision in poor light, eyeache, headache, local irritation
   b. Systemic: flushing, diaphoresis, GI upset, diarrhea
4. Drug examples
   a. Cholinergics: pilocarpine (Isopto Carpine), carbachol (Miostat)
   b. Cholinesterase inhibitors: demecarium bromide (Humorsol)

G. Beta-adrenergic blocking agents: specific information
1. Indications: open-angle glaucoma; topical medication
2. Side effects: ocular irritation, visual disturbances
3. Drug example: timolol maleate (Timoptic)

H. Carbonic anhydrase inhibitors: specific information
1. Indications: open-angle and narrow-angle glaucoma; systemic medication
2. Side effects: lethargy, anorexia, drowsiness, depression, malaise, diuresis, numbness and tingling of extremities
3. Drug example: acetazolamide (Diamox)

I. Osmotic diuretics (see Section XVI): specific information
1. Indications: preoperative and postoperative short-term reduction of intraocular pressure; systemic medication
2. Side effects: headache, nausea, vomiting, thirst, diarrhea, agitation, disorientation, convulsions, CHF
3. Drug examples
   a. Mannitol (Osmitrol)
   b. Glycerin (Glyrol)

J. Mydriatics and cycloplegics: specific information
1. Mechanism of action
   a. Anticholinergics inhibit the parasympathetic nervous system and cause mydriasis and cycloplegia
   b. Adrenergics mimic the actions of the sympathetic nervous system and cause mydriasis

2. Indications
   a. Eye examinations
   b. Inflammatory eye conditions
   c. Prevention of adhesions
   d. Preparation for surgery
3. Side effects
   a. Ocular: increased intraocular pressure, eyeache, headache, hypersensitivity, photophobia
   b. Systemic: tachycardia, hypertension, dry mouth
4. Patient teaching: tell patient that he may need to wear dark glasses following eye examination to prevent photophobia
5. Drug examples
   a. Anticholinergics: atropine sulfate (BufOpto Atropine), cyclopentolate (Cyclogyl), tropicamide (Mydriacyl)
   b. Adrenergics: epinephrine (Epitrate), phenylephrine hydrochloride (Neo-Synephrine)

Points to Remember

Topical glaucoma medications work by opening the anterior chamber angle and increasing the outflow, or decreasing aqueous humor production.

Systemic medications for glaucoma decrease aqueous humor production or decrease the intraocular pressure by increasing the intravascular osmotic pressure, thus creating an osmotic gradient that pulls fluid from the eye.

The patient with glaucoma should carry identification describing the disease and drug therapy.

An eye patch may be necessary to protect the eye from injury until the corneal reflex returns when a patient receives an anesthetic for the eye.

Glossary

Accommodation—adjustment of the eye by contraction of the ciliary muscles and change in the lens curvature that allows focusing at various distances. Cycloplegics paralyze the ciliary muscles and inhibit accommodation

Corneal reflex—closure of the eyelids upon direct touch or irritation of the eye. This reflex is lost when corneal anesthetics are used

Mydriasis—dilation of the pupil

Myopia—a defect in vision in which objects can be seen distinctly only when close to the eyes; nearsightedness

Nonpyogenic—without pus production

The Patient with an Ear Disorder

Learning Objectives

After studying this section, the reader should be able to:

● Describe the mechanism of action of the various drugs used to treat ear disorders.

● List common side effects of drugs used to treat ear disorders.

● Identify the nursing implications during assessment, implementation, and evaluation of the patient receiving drugs used to treat ear disorders.

● Describe the correct technique for instilling ear drops in adults and in children.

● Discuss appropriate patient teaching for the patient receiving drugs used to treat ear disorders.

XL. The Patient with an Ear Disorder

A. **Drugs for ear disorders: general information**
   1. Mechanism of action
      a. Anti-infectives kill or inhibit the growth of susceptible bacteria
      b. Antihistamines and decongestants reduce ear effusion
      c. Local anesthetics control pain associated with ear infections
      d. Cerumenolytic agents soften, loosen, and flush out deposits of cerumen
   2. Indications: see specific information
   3. Contraindications: hypersensitivity
   4. Interactions: none significant
   5. Nursing implications
      a. Assessment: assess patient for hearing loss, pain, and drainage
      b. Implementation: use correct method for instillation of ear drops for adults and children. Pull down on the auricle to straighten external canal in a child. Pull up and back on the auricle to straighten the external canal of an adult
      c. Evaluation: base on resolution of signs and symptoms of ear disorder
   6. Patient teaching: instruct patient in the correct administration procedure

C. **Anti-infectives (see Section XXVIII): specific information**
   1. Indications: otitis media or externa
   2. Drug examples
      a. Polymixin B (Aerosporin, Otobiotic, Neosporin)
      b. Chloramphenicol (Cholormycetin)
      c. Ampicillin (Polycillin, Omnipen, Amcill)
      d. Sulfamethoxazole/trimethoprim (Septra, Bactrim)
      e. Penicillin (Pentids, V-Cillin, Pen-Vee)
      f. Amoxicillin (Amoxil, Larotid, Polymox)
      g. Cefaclor (Ceclor)

D. **Antihistamines and decongestants: specific information**
   1. Indications: adjunctive therapy for acute otitis media
   2. Drug examples: antihistamine-decongestant combinations (Actifed, Allerest, Chlor-Trimeton, Dimetane, Drixoral, Novahistine, Triaminic)

E. **Local anesthetics: specific information**
   1. Indications: pain associated with ear infections
   2. Drug examples: benzocaine (Americaine-Otic, Tympagesic)

F. **Ceruminolytic agents: specific information**
   1. Indications: removal of excess cerumen; efficacy compared to olive oil, glycerin, or hydrogen peroxide is questionable
   2. Drug examples
      a. Triethanolamine polypeptide oleate-condensate (Cerumenex)
      b. Carbamide peroxide (Debrox)

Points to Remember

Antihistamines and decongestants reduce nasal congestion and ear effusion.

To instill eardrops in an adult, the auricle should be pulled up and back to straighten the external canal.

To instill eardrops in a child, the auricle should be pulled down.

The efficacy of cerumenolytic agents is questionable compared to olive oil, glycerin, or hydrogen peroxide.

Glossary

Auricle—external ear

Cerumen—earwax

Otitis externa—infection or inflammation of external ear canal or auricle

Otitis media—infection or inflammation of middle ear

The Patient with a Skin Disorder

Learning Objectives

After studying this section, the reader should be able to:

● Describe the mechanism of action of the various drugs used to treat skin disorders.

● List common side effects of drugs used to treat skin disorders.

● Identify the nursing implications during assessment, implementation, and evaluation of the patient receiving drugs used to treat skin disorders.

● Discuss appropriate patient teaching for the patient receiving drugs used to treat skin disorders.

XLI. The Patient with a Skin Disorder

A. Drugs for skin disorders: general information
1. Mechanism of action
   a. Emollients allow skin to retain water
   b. Keratolytics break down protein in keratin
   c. Antibacterial agents kill or inhibit the growth of susceptible bacteria
   d. Antifungal agents kill or inhibit the growth of susceptible fungi
   e. Antiviral agents kill or inhibit the growth of susceptible viruses
   f. Antiparasitic agents kill parasitic arthropods
   g. Anti-inflammatory agents decrease inflammation, itching, and cause vasoconstriction
   h. Debriding agents digest necrotic collagenous tissue
   i. Antipruritics relieve itching of skin and mucous membranes
   j. Acne products clean and dry the skin (cleanser/antiseptics), reduce bacteria that cause infection (antibiotics), or reduce the size and activity of sebaceous glands (isotretinoin)
2. Indications: see specific information
3. Contraindications: hypersensitivity
4. Side effects: skin irritation
5. Interactions: none significant
6. Nursing implications
   a. Assessment: assess skin lesions for spreading or healing
   b. Implementation: remove old medication from the skin before each application. Aseptic technique is necessary for application to open lesions. Psychological support may be important to the patient with a skin disorder
   c. Evaluation: base on resolution of skin lesions
7. Patient teaching: instruct patient on correct technique for application of medication

B. Emollients: specific information
1. Indications: treatment of dry skin
2. Drug examples
   a. Cold cream
   b. Zinc ointment

C. Keratolytics: specific information
1. Indications: superficial fungal infections, psoriasis, seborrheic dermatitis, corns, and callouses
2. Drug examples
   a. Salicylic acid
   b. Resorcinol

D. Antibacterial agents: specific information
  1. Indications: bacterial skin infections
  2. Drug examples
     a. Bacitracin
     b. Neosporin G (neomycin, polymixin B, gramicidin)
     c. Polysporin (zinc bacitracin, polymixin B)

E. Antifungal agents (see Section XXX): specific information
  1. Indications: fungal skin infections
  2. Drug examples
     a. Miconazole (Monistat)
     b. Clotrimazole (Lotrimin, Mycelex)
     c. Ketoconazole (Nizoral)
     d. Griseofulvin (Fulvicin, Grifulvin, Grisactin)

F. Antiviral agents (see Section XXXI): specific information
  1. Indications: herpes simplex types 1 and 2
  2. Drug example: acyclovir (Zovirax)

G. Antiparasitic agents: specific information
  1. Indications: scabies (mites) or pediculosis (lice)
  2. Drug example: lindane (Kwell)

H. Anti-inflammatory agents (see Section XXIII): specific information
  1. Indications: dermatitis, allergic skin reactions
  2. Side effects: potential for systemic side effects if used in large quantities and absorbed
  3. Drug examples
     a. Hydrocortisone (Cort-Dome)
     b. Triamcinalone (Kenolog, Aristocort)
     c. Dexamethasone (Decadron, Decaderm)
     d. Coal-tar preparations

I. Debriding agents: specific information
  1. Indications: decubiti and burns
  2. Drug examples
     a. Sutilains (Travase)
     b. Fibrinolysin and deoxyribonucleic acid (Elase)
     c. Dextranomer (Debrisan)

J. Antipruritic agents: specific information
  1. Indications: pruritus
  2. Drug examples
     a. Oatmeal baths (Aveeno)
     b. Calamine lotion
     c. Diphenhydramine (Benadryl)
     d. Cyproheptadine (Periactin)

K. Acne products: specific information
1. Indications
    a. Acne vulgaris (cleanser/antiseptics, antibiotics)
    b. Cystic acne vulgaris (isotretinoin)
2. Contraindications: pregnancy and lactation (isotretinoin)
3. Side effects: burning, redness, or itching of the eyes, nosebleeds, scaling, redness, burning or pain of the lips, and photosensitivity (isotretinoin)
4. Patient teaching
    a. Tell patient taking isotretinoin to use sunscreen and protective clothing to prevent photosensitivity reactions
    b. Tell patient taking isotretinoin to use contraception and not to give blood during or within 30 days after therapy to prevent the possibility of pregnant women receiving the blood
5. Drug examples
    a. Cleanser/antiseptics: benzoyl peroxide
    b. Antibiotics: clindamycin (Cleocin T topical solution), erythromycin (EryDerm), tetracycline (Topicycline)
    c. Isotretinoin (Accutane)

Points to Remember

Emollients allow the skin to retain water.

Keratolytics break down protein in keratin.

Debriding agents digest necrotic collagenous tissue.

Before administering topical medications for skin disorders, skin lesions should be assessed and old medication removed.

Glossary

Debride—to remove foreign material and dead or damaged tissue from wounds or burns

Decubiti—inflammation, sore, or ulcers in the skin resulting from tissue ischemia, commonly called bedsores

Keratin—protein that is the main constituent of the epidermis, hair, and nails

Necrotic—relating to localized tissue death

Index